LASIK
THE EYE LASER
MIRACLE

LASIK

THE EYE LASER MIRACLE

THE COMPLETE GUIDE
TO BETTER VISION

ANDREW I. CASTER, M.D., F.A.C.S.

BALLANTINE BOOKS

NEW YORK

||||||||||||||||||||||||||||||||||||||||||||||||||||||||||||||||||||||||||||||

The advice, information, and guidelines
presented in this book are not intended to replace
professional medical advice. All care and treatment of your
eyes should be administered by an eye care professional.

CONTENTS

PART II

ADDITIONAL INFORMATION—

FOR THOSE WHO WANT TO KNOW MORE

AFTERWORD

APPENDIXES

INTRODUCTION

Seeing well without glasses and contact lenses is the dream of millions of Americans. Modern medical science has enabled this dream to come true.

Laser vision correction is the extremely popular treatment for nearsightedness, farsightedness, and astigmatism, and it can permanently eliminate the need to wear glasses or contact lenses for distance vision. The most common version of laser vision correction, Lasik (laser in-situ keratomileusis), uses an invisible laser beam to reshape the inner layers of the cornea (the clear, curved structure at the front of the eye).

Another version of laser vision correction, known as PRK (photorefractive keratectomy) or Advanced Surface Treatment, applies the laser treatment to the outer portion of the cornea. Both versions of laser vision correction are very quick—usually taking only about five minutes—and painless. The results, as patients and their doctors will tell you, are impressive.

• Stacy, a forty-year-old music publisher, had been wearing corrective lenses since she was in the sixth grade. For thirty years, she couldn't get out of bed in the morning without putting on her glasses. "As a child, I would play a game: If I had three wishes, what would they be? 20/20 vision, 20/20 vision, 20/20 vision. It's always been the first thing I would change about my life." Three weeks after having Lasik, Stacy's vision had improved from 20/800 to 20/20. "Your confidence level goes up," she said. "It's not so much the way you look. It's the way you feel. I feel so good about myself."

• Ted was so nearsighted and astigmatic that he could barely see his hand in front of his face without glasses. Before having surgery, he went sailing with his nine-year-old son. The boom knocked Ted's glasses off. He grabbed them just before they landed in the water. Without them, he couldn't see the shore. That close call convinced him that it was time to get rid of his glasses. Lasik surgery gave him 20/25 vision. "What's dramatic," the forty-eight-year-old teacher said, "is being able to open your eyes in the morning and actually being able to see."

• Ethan, a thirty-two-year-old actor with 20/800 vision, had been wearing contact lenses for years. By the end of the day, his eyes were tired and red. Now that he's had PRK, he has 20/25 vision in the left eye and 20/20 in the right. "It's one less worry in my life," he said. "It's made my life a little less complicated. I don't have to put in contacts or get my glasses. I just feel freer."

• Lasik treatment gave Diane, a forty-five-year-old physician's assistant, a newfound sense of freedom, too. Before Lasik, she couldn't clearly see her feet when she was in the shower. Now she's taking rock-climbing lessons with her twelve-year-old daughter, something she would never do when she had to wear glasses or contacts. "I always believed I was entitled to see well," she said. With 20/30 vision in her left eye and 20/40 in her right, she finally does. "It's within a person's grasp. It's wonderful that technology has come this far."

Because of the ease of treatment and the accuracy of results, laser vision correction has become one of the most commonly performed surgeries in the United States. More than one million laser vision correction procedures are performed each year in the United States, and a similar number in the rest of the world.

However, laser vision correction is not for everyone, and it is not risk free. It is also not 100 percent effective for all patients.

I have written this book to explain to you the pros and cons of laser vision correction and to present other information necessary to help you make an informed decision. Part I provides basic information and should be read by everyone contemplating this procedure, Part II provides additional information for those who want to know more, and the Afterword describes my own experience as a patient having laser vision correction. Part I includes simple background information, the characteristics of a good candidate for laser vision treatment, and how the procedure works. Part I also describes the procedure itself, from the presurgical consultation through the postoperative phase. Finally, it points out what results you can expect and what can go wrong. The last section of Part I answers the most commonly asked questions about laser vision correction. All readers will find this particularly useful.

Part II is for people who desire additional information, a behind-the-scenes exploration. It describes what a laser is, the role of the FDA in evaluating the laser procedure, alternatives to laser vision treatment, as well as possible future developments.

This book provides the consumer with important background information concerning laser vision correction. Every effort has been made to provide accurate information and a balanced viewpoint, but the accuracy of information cannot be guaranteed. When statistics are given, they are usually taken from FDA supervised studies, but multiple studies conducted in different fashions produce varying statistics. The decision to have laser vision correction must be based upon an evaluation and critical discussion with your doctor of your specific medical condition, lifestyle, and desires.

PART
I

||||||||||||||||||||||||||||

BASIC
INFORMATION

—

EVERYONE
SHOULD READ
THIS

||||||||||||||||||||||||||

THE

TREATMENT IS EASY

Laser vision correction is a very easy procedure to undergo. No injections are needed, and there is no pain during the procedure. These are the steps you will experience:

1. Your doctor will measure your eyes to determine your amount of nearsightedness, farsightedness, and astigmatism. During this presurgical consultation, your doctor will complete a thorough examination of the health of your eyes and discuss the procedure in detail with you.

2. The laser will be calibrated and tested for accuracy.

3. The correction desired for your eye will be entered into the laser's computer.

4. The computer will determine the specific set of laser pulses to apply.

5. You will be brought into the laser room and asked to lie down.

6. A patch will be placed over the eye not having the procedure.

7. Anesthetic eyedrops will be placed in the eye. No injections or IVs are needed.

8. Your eyelid will be held open with a small speculum, which causes no pain.

9. You will be asked to look at a small blinking light.

10. In Lasik, a small layer of tissue, known as the corneal flap, will be separated and lifted. In PRK, the doctor will gently wipe away the soft, superficial layer covering the cornea.

11. You will hear a clicking noise, the sound of the laser.

12. The blinking light will get hazy as the treatment progresses.

13. The treatment will usually take less than thirty seconds of laser time.

14. Eyedrops will be placed in the eye. In some cases, a temporary contact lens will be placed in the eye as well.

15. In most cases, the procedure will then be repeated for the second eye.

16. You will sit up and rest for a few minutes before going home. Your stay in the treatment room has lasted about five to ten minutes.

Sounds easy, doesn't it? And it is. But how accurate are the results? What can go wrong? Are you a suitable candidate for laser vision correction, or should you consider alternatives? These questions will be addressed shortly. First, we will examine the mechanics of the eye.

HOW DOES

THE EYE WORK?

Just like a camera, the eye works by focusing light rays. Light entering the eye first passes through a transparent layer called the cornea. The cornea acts as a lens by focusing the light. Located behind the cornea is another lens, known as the crystalline lens, that further focuses the light to make a clear image on the retina at the back of the eye. Finally, the image is transmitted to the brain by the optic nerve.

Just as a camera cannot produce a clear photograph if the incoming light is not focused precisely onto the back of the camera, so the eye cannot produce clear vision if the cornea and crystalline lens do not focus the light precisely onto the retina.

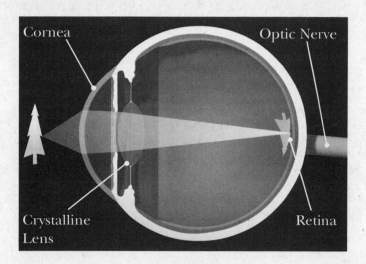

The eye is very similar to a camera. Light rays are focused by the cornea and crystalline lens. The focus must be accurate in order to obtain a clear image.

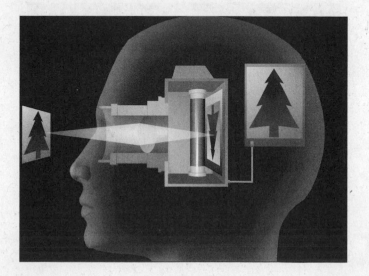

COMMON
VISION PROBLEMS

The most common vision problem is the inability to focus incoming light precisely onto the retina. The result is blurred vision.

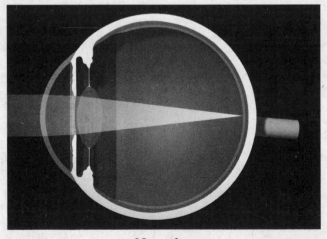

Normal eye

There are four types of focusing errors:

Nearsightedness. Nearsighted people see near objects more clearly than objects farther away. In nearsightedness (also known as myopia), light rays from distant objects are focused not onto the retina but in front of the retina. Nearsightedness occurs because the cornea and the crystalline lens together have too much focusing power for the length of the eye. If the cornea and the crystalline lens had less combined focusing power, or if the eye were shorter, then the light rays would be focused precisely onto the retina.

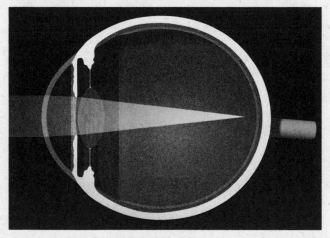

Nearsighted eye

Farsightedness. Farsighted people see faraway objects more clearly than they see nearby objects. In mild cases of farsightedness, or in younger people, only near objects will be blurry. In moderate cases, or in older individuals, both far and near vision will be blurry, but the near vision will be more affected. Farsightedness (also known as hyperopia) results when the cornea and crystalline lens together have too little focusing power for the length of the eye. Light rays from distant objects are focused not onto the retina but behind the retina. If the cornea and the crystalline lens had more combined focusing power, or if the eye were longer, then the light rays would be focused precisely onto the retina.

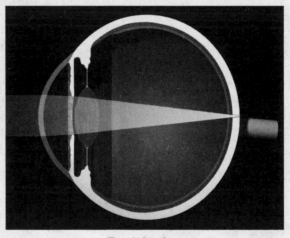

Farsighted eye

Astigmatism. People whose eyes focus light rays unevenly have astigmatism. Astigmatism occurs when the cornea has an irregular shape. The cornea should be round and symmetrical like a basketball, but in cases of astigmatism it is shaped more like a football or the back of a spoon. People with astigmatism see both near and far objects out of focus. Astigmatism frequently accompanies nearsightedness or farsightedness.

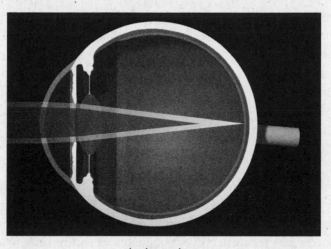

Astigmatic eye

Presbyopia. Presbyopia (which comes from the Greek for "old vision") refers to the gradual loss, as we age, of the eye's ability to adjust the focus from far to near. Presbyopia is a normal part of the aging process, affecting each and every person, and usually begins to cause a problem with near vision between the ages of forty and fifty. It is corrected by the use of reading glasses or bifocals. Presbyopia occurs because the crystalline lens no longer adequately adjusts its shape to focus clearly on close-up objects.

Presbyopia is referred to as "farsightedness" by most people and is frequently confused with true farsightedness (hyperopia). Presbyopia and hyperopia are often confused because both compromise up-close vision, though in entirely different ways. Presbyopia is an age-related loss of flexibility of the crystalline lens. Hyperopia is caused by too little focusing power in the eye—a combination of the cornea, the crystalline lens, and the length of the eye. Whereas presbyopia is an aging effect that begins to be experienced sometime after thirty-five years of age, hyperopia affects people of all ages, even young children.

Presbyopia can be present by itself or in combination with nearsightedness, farsightedness, or astigmatism.

In ancient times, people with focusing errors had to live with blurry vision. During the late Middle Ages (around A.D. 1250), the first glasses were developed. For almost seven hundred years, glasses were the only treatment available for focusing errors. In the 1930s, hard contact lenses were developed, followed in the 1970s by soft contacts.

Glasses and contact lenses improve vision by helping the eye to focus the incoming light rays. They subtract focusing power from nearsighted eyes and add focusing power to farsighted eyes. Bifocal lenses help people with presbyopia to see faraway objects (through the upper portion) as well as near objects (through the lower portion).

||||||||||||||||||||||||||||||

HOW DOES
LASER TREATMENT
IMPROVE VISION?

A laser is a device that creates a very special kind of light energy. The light can be of any color and can be invisible to the human eye.

The excimer laser makes pulses of invisible ultraviolet light. Each pulse of light removes a microscopically thin layer from the cornea, changing the curvature of the cornea ever so slightly. A computer running specialized software determines the exact pattern of pulses needed to remove the right amount of corneal tissue.

To correct nearsightedness, the curvature of the cornea must be decreased—the cornea must be made flatter. Tissue is removed in a disc-shaped pattern, with more tissue removed from the center than the edges. To correct farsightedness, the central portion of the cornea must be made steeper. This is accomplished by removing tissue in a doughnut-shaped pattern. To correct astigmatism, the cornea must be made more symmetrical.

The laser pulses may be applied to the surface of the cornea, in which case the treatment is known as PRK. Alternatively, the laser treatment may be applied to the deeper portion of the cornea, under a thin layer of tissue; this variation is known as Lasik.

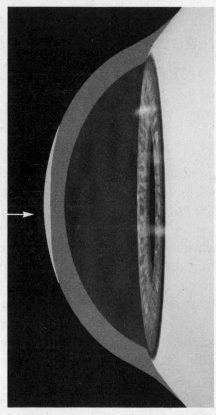

To correct nearsightedness, farsightedness, and astigmatism, the laser removes a small amount of tissue (see arrow) from the cornea, causing the shape of the cornea to change ever so slightly.

Only a very small amount of tissue is removed, usually less than the width of a hair. Mild focusing problems will require small amounts of tissue removal. Severe focusing errors will require greater amounts of tissue removal. The total treatment usually takes less than thirty seconds of actual laser time.

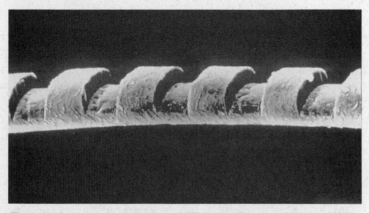

Excimer lasers are very precise! This is a human hair etched by an excimer laser.

||||||||||||||||||||||||||||

ARE YOU
A GOOD CANDIDATE?

Some people should definitely not have laser vision correction. These include:

• People who are very happy wearing glasses or contact lenses. They have no need for the procedure.

• People under eighteen years old. Their focusing error is probably still increasing. But there is no upper age limit for laser vision treatment.

• People whose vision is significantly changing. Glasses or contact lens prescriptions often continue to change through the teenage years into the early twenties. At least two years should pass without a significant change. (A significant change is one half diopter or more.)

• People who insist upon a perfect correction. A perfect correction is possible but cannot be guaranteed.

- Women who are pregnant or who are breast-feeding. Hormonal changes will often cause temporary changes in nearsightedness, farsightedness, or astigmatism.

You should consider this procedure, first of all, if you are not in any of the above categories. Second, you must have nearsightedness, farsightedness, or astigmatism. You may have presbyopia as well, but presbyopia cannot currently be corrected with laser vision correction, except through a technique known as monovision (see the chapter titled "If You Are Over Thirty-five"). Third, you must want to be free of your glasses or contact lenses to the extent that you are willing to invest the time, energy, and money to understand and undergo the procedure. Even then, not everyone who wants to have the procedure will be able to, at least not now.

IIIIIIIIIIIIIIIIIIIIIIIIIIIII

THE PRETREATMENT
CONSULTATION

The pretreatment consultation is a very important part of the laser vision correction process. You can expect the following issues to be addressed during the pretreatment consultation, and it is important that you are comfortable with the resolution of each issue.

Refraction. The doctor must determine whether you are a suitable candidate for the procedure. This depends on a variety of factors, including your age and occupation, but the doctor will be concerned primarily with your refractive (focusing) error—that is, your ideal glasses or contact lens prescription. The doctor's recommendation to proceed or not will depend on an assessment of all the factors. An initial consultation may be scheduled to determine if you are a good candidate, with final measurements taken at a later consultation. If you wear soft lenses, you will need to stop wearing them at least one week before the final consultation; if you wear hard or gas-permeable lenses, stop wearing them at least six weeks before the final consultation. This is very important, because contact lenses can temporarily alter the shape of the cornea and the natural shape of your cornea must be accurately determined prior to the treatment.

Complete Examination. Your doctor will perform a complete eye examination to determine the overall health of your eyes. Certain eye conditions may make you less suitable, or even ineligible, for the procedure. Included in this examination should be several tests, all of which are entirely painless, including a computer-assisted measurement of the contours of your cornea, known as corneal topography, a measurement of your pupil size in the dark, a measurement of the thickness of your cornea, and a wavefront measurement of the distortions in your vision. (For more details on these tests, please read "Five Important Tests—and What They Mean.")

When Claire, a fifty-three-year-old photographer, had her topography done, she rested her chin on a metal bar and stared for a few seconds into a concave dome covered with concentric black-and-white lines similar to a target. She stared into the dome for a few seconds with one eye and then with the other. "You don't touch anything, and it doesn't touch you," Claire explained. A minute later, a computer on the other side of the dome printed out a topographical map of the shape of her cornea, showing how steep it was from point to point.

Doctor's Experience and Bedside Manner. You should meet the surgeon and make sure that you feel very comfortable with his or her education, bedside manner, and refractive surgery experience. Is the doctor board certified in ophthalmology? How long has the doctor been performing laser vision surgery? How many Lasik or PRK procedures has he or she performed? How many procedures does the doctor perform each week? Does the doctor enjoy a good reputation in the community? You need to have complete confidence in the surgeon who will perform the procedure.

Pros, Cons, and Alternatives. The advantages, disadvantages, and alternatives to laser vision correction must be thoroughly discussed. What are the chances of actually achieving your desired results—good vision without glasses or contact lenses? Be sure to understand what problems might arise. And remember that nonsurgical treatments—glasses or contact lenses—always remain an option.

Informed Consent. You will be asked to sign papers confirming that you understand the risks and benefits of, and alternatives to, laser vision correction. These papers may contain words or ideas that you do not understand. Consider taking the papers home for slow, careful review before signing them. Also consider having a relative or friend review the papers to help you better understand them. Do not sign the papers until you completely understand all the words and concepts. These papers are legally binding and are designed to ensure that you understand the important aspects of the procedure. You do not have to sign the papers at the time of your initial consultation, although you cannot undergo the treatment until you do sign them.

Costs. All financial arrangements should be openly discussed. Often the fee can be paid by credit card, or your doctor may have a financing plan. Beware of fees that are unusually high or low. The fees for this procedure are not regulated in any way. Abnormally low fees raise questions of quality, and abnormally high fees may not be justified.

If you don't know anyone who has had laser vision treatment, ask the doctor to put you in touch with a few patients. Stacy decided to have Lasik after a friend who had undergone the procedure described it to her in detail. The personal testimonial made all the difference. "She told me everything I would be feeling," Stacy said. "It really helps talking to someone who's had it done. A doctor can tell you the technical stuff, but hearing it from someone who's been through it is a lot different."

||||||||||||||||||||||||||||

FLAP OR NO FLAP?

The most popular version of laser vision correction is called Lasik (laser in-situ keratomileusis). In Lasik, a very thin layer of tissue in the front of the cornea, known as a flap, is separated and folded out of the way. The laser treatment is then applied to the deeper part of the cornea beneath the flap. The flap, which remains attached at one edge, is then folded back into place and quickly heals. Think of the flap as a protective "Band-Aid."

The other common version of laser vision correction is known as PRK (photorefractive keratectomy) or Advanced Surface Treatment. With slight variations it is also known as epi-Lasik and Lasek. In PRK, the laser energy is applied to the surface of the cornea, so no creation of a flap is required. PRK is essentially "Lasik without a flap."

When the laser treatment is applied to the tissue deep within the cornea instead of to the surface, the vi-

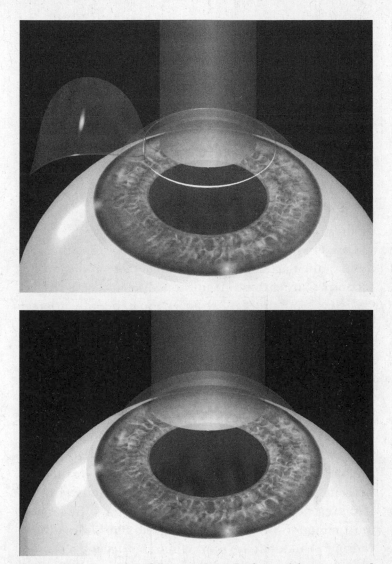

In Lasik (top), a thin flap is made in the front of the cornea and the laser treatment is performed on the deeper cornea. In PRK (bottom), the laser energy is applied to the surface of the cornea.

sion recovery is quicker. Patients usually see very well the day after Lasik. With PRK, the vision is useful right away, but takes longer to become extremely sharp.

Neither Lasik nor PRK involves any pain during the procedure, but Lasik patients experience less posttreatment discomfort. Most of the pain fibers in the cornea are in the surface portion. In Lasik, the surface of the cornea is not treated, so very few pain fibers are affected. Most Lasik patients take no pain medicine after the procedure. In PRK, there is more discomfort after the treatment. This discomfort is controlled by the use of anesthetic eyedrops for several days.

Lasik requires an additional surgical step, the creation of the flap. Creation of the flap takes about twenty seconds. During this time, most people have a feeling of "pressure" on the eye, though some people do feel slight pain. After the treatment is complete, the flap is pushed back into its original position. No stitches are used, because the flap is held in position by natural corneal suction.

For most patients, the creation of the flap is the most worrisome aspect of laser vision treatment. These flaps have been created for other eye procedures for over thirty years. Difficulties can occur with the flap, but in the hands of an experienced surgeon occur less than 1 percent of the time. Most of the complications with the flap are mild and resolve within a few days. By far the most common problem is having the flap slide a little, causing wrinkles in the flap. When this occurs, it is most typically during the first day after the procedure, before the flap has had a chance to firmly set into position, and is corrected by lifting and repositioning the flap. Improper creation of the flap, resulting in an irregularity in the flap, is the most serious complication. When this occurs, which is less than 1 percent of the time, the patient will be asked to wait several months, and the treatment will then be completed without a flap.

Most people choose the Lasik version of the procedure because of the extremely rapid vision recovery and minimal posttreatment pain. However, some people are not good candidates for Lasik, but are suitable for PRK. These would include people with very thin corneas, people with hobbies or occupations (such as boxing) where there is a good likelihood they will be hit in the eye, or people with specific, unusual conditions of the cornea. Although these patients might prefer to have Lasik, the PRK procedure would be a better choice. The decision of which technique is best in your situation must be made by you and your doctor.

WHAT DOES
CUSTOM WAVEFRONT
TREATMENT MEAN?

The most significant focusing abnormalities of the eye are nearsightedness, farsightedness, and astigmatism. In addition, the eye has other, more subtle irregularities, known as higher order aberrations, which glasses and contact lenses are not able to correct. If these aberrations are large, they can affect the quality of the vision, particularly in low contrast or low light levels.

When a laser treatment adjusts for higher order aberrations in addition to nearsightedness, farsightedness, and astigmatism, it is called a "custom" treatment. The measurement of these aberrations is known as "wavefront." With custom wavefront treatments, two people with the same glasses prescription will receive slightly different laser treatments, in order to adjust for the higher order aberrations.

Because custom treatments can correct imperfections in the vision that glasses and contacts cannot correct, many people who have custom laser treatment actually see better without contacts or glasses after the treatment than they saw before the laser treatment with their glasses or contacts. "I am really shocked," explains Richard, a thirty-five-year-old marketing representative. "I never liked my contacts, because they weren't very comfortable. But I always thought I could see pretty well. But now I am seeing leaves and all sorts of other things that I could never see before. It is truly amazing!"

Custom wavefront treatments are performed with both the Lasik and PRK techniques—both with and without a flap. From the patient's viewpoint, the treatment experience is identical for custom and non-custom procedures. But on average, custom treatments produce slightly better vision than non-custom treatments. Often, the improvement in vision resulting from custom wavefront treatment is most significant in the most difficult viewing circumstances, such as low contrast or low light levels.

||||||||||||||||||||||||||||

THE TREATMENT EXPERIENCE:
THE PATIENT'S PERSPECTIVE

What is it like to have Lasik or PRK? Does it hurt? Is it frightening? Will it take a long time to recover? Do the benefits outweigh the risks?

Bruce, a forty-year-old accountant with 20/800 vision, was asking himself those questions as he sat in the waiting room on the morning of his treatment. He had been wearing glasses since the first grade. Without them, he was so nearsighted that he couldn't read the alarm clock from bed.

For years he had tried contact lenses, but he could never wear them for long. Within a few hours, wind and dust would leave his eyes red and teary. And he hated the hassle of caring for his lenses—the chemicals, the cleanings, the midnight runs to the drugstore for saline, and the constant worries about dropping a contact or having one get lost in his eye.

Glasses weren't much better. "I go swimming with my children and take my glasses off, and I can't find my kids in the pool," he said. "I'm always fearful that I'll lose my glasses, and I won't be able to see. Peripheral vision is nonexistent, and for playing sports, that's important. I play basketball, ride my bike to work, horse around with the kids, coach the softball team. I don't want to over-play it, but in a certain way, it's a handicap."

Melanie, a twenty-six-year-old lobbyist, felt the same way. Like Bruce, she had been wearing corrective lenses since grammar school, switching back and forth be-tween glasses and contacts. She had nearsightedness so severe, she said, that it left her "totally reliant on glasses or contact lenses for everything. If I knocked my glasses off my bed stand, I was helpless, crawling around on the floor trying to find them by feel. It drove me crazy. I felt so vulnerable."

Bruce decided to have PRK performed on his eyes. Melanie opted for Lasik. Before the procedure, they had complete eye exams. They read the eye chart, looked through different lenses, and had corneal topographies. Both were good candidates for laser vision correction.

Still, as he sat in the waiting room, Bruce wondered if he was doing the right thing. "I'm a conservative, nerdy accountant watching my livelihood possibly going out the window. Not to mention seeing my family for the last time. The reality is that I'm probably more likely to get hit by a car riding home on my bike than I am to have something seriously go wrong with this procedure. You don't think about getting hit by a car when you ride your bike. But this is like, 'Okay, lie back, here it comes. Look at the red light.' "

Melanie had some preoperative jitters, too. "It was a little scary, because Lasik seems more invasive than

PRK," she said. "With PRK, there's no cutting of your eye and lifting it up. The flap was probably the one thing that made me the most nervous. I worried about what would happen if the flap didn't get back on the right way."

About twenty minutes before the treatment, a nurse will administer a combination of anti-inflammatory and anesthetic drops into the patient's eyes. Both PRK and Lasik are performed with local anesthetic eyedrops. No other medication—injected, intravenous, or oral—is needed, although doctors often give patients Xanax or Valium to calm their nerves. Melanie took a Valium while sitting in the waiting room. Her legs felt a little wobbly as she walked into the laser treatment room.

The setting for laser vision correction is anything but surgical. Both Bruce and Melanie wore their street clothes. Other than a computer, some chairs, and the laser itself, which is about seven feet long, the room is empty. Before a PRK or Lasik patient enters the room, a technician programs the laser's computer to provide the exact set of laser pulses needed to correct his or her refractive error.

Bruce sat in a reclining chair, similar to the kind found in a dentist's office, and the doctor positioned him under the laser. The doctor put a U-shaped pillow around Bruce's head to keep him from moving and placed an eye patch over his left eye. He then put a small metal speculum, also known as a retractor, around Bruce's right eye to hold the eyelid open.

Up to this point, Melanie's experience was identical to Bruce's. She sat in the same chair with a pillow placed around her neck. The doctor covered one of her eyes and put a speculum around the eyelid of the other eye. Melanie had been dreading the speculum. "I suspected that it would be the worst part of the procedure and that it would hurt, but it wasn't really that noticeable. You could feel someone touching and moving your eyelid a little bit away from your eye, but there was no pain." Although Melanie couldn't close her eye, she could move it in any direction.

The primary differences between PRK and Lasik occur at the beginning and end of the procedures. For Bruce's PRK, the doctor put the speculum around Bruce's eyelid and then used a small instrument to wipe away the epithelium, the soft, most superficial layer of the cornea. Bruce could see a shadow passing across his eye, but all he felt was a little bit of pressure. There wasn't any pain, and it took only a few seconds for the doctor to finish. Some doctors use the laser itself to remove the epithelium during PRK; others believe that manual or chemical removal is preferable.

For a Lasik patient like Melanie, the doctor needed to create a thin flap within the front of her cornea that could be peeled back to reveal the tissue underneath. Melanie stared at a small light overhead and felt some pressure on her eye. It took only a few seconds to make the flap and fold it back. "When the flap was actually being lifted up, it was blurry for a moment," Melanie recalled. "I remember thinking what a strange sensation it was, but none of it hurt."

The laser portion of the surgery is similar for PRK and Lasik patients. The doctor told Bruce to lie still, to focus on the blinking light, and to relax. "Crisscross apprehension with nervousness, with excitement, with fear of the unknown—that's what I was feeling," Bruce said. But the doctor talked Bruce through the treatment, explaining to him exactly what would happen at each stage. Bruce heard the laser make a series of loud clicking noises, akin to a bug zapper, and he caught a whiff of something that smelled like singed hair. He felt no pain, and less than thirty seconds later, the laser stopped firing.

Like Bruce, Melanie had less than a minute of laser time. She noticed that as the laser sequence progressed, the red light on which she was focusing changed. "At the beginning, I couldn't even pinpoint where the light was. It was just a blur. But as they used the laser, I could tell my vision was getting better. It was a little sharper."

After completing the laser treatment on Melanie's eye, the doctor flushed it out with water—a strange sensation, Melanie remembered, because she could see the water being sprayed across her eye and could feel it trickling down the side of her face but could not feel it on her anesthetized eye.

Once the laser sequence ends, PRK and Lasik patients have slightly different experiences. When Bruce's treatment was over, the doctor put some drops in his eye, including an antibiotic to prevent infection and an anti-inflammatory medication to minimize discomfort. He then placed a clear contact lens in Bruce's eye to protect the cornea and decrease pain. Bruce sat up and looked across the room. There was an assistant standing a few feet away and, despite the fact that the contact lens made his vision somewhat cloudy, Bruce could read the man's name tag. "A total sense of euphoria came over me," Bruce remembered. "I wasn't blind, and the bonus was that I could really see."

After the doctor finished treating Melanie's eye, he pushed the corneal flap back into its original position. Melanie experienced a momentary blurriness as he repositioned the tissue. The doctor put some drops in her eye. Then she looked up at his assistants. "I remember seeing them right away. For about three feet out, I could see really well, whereas before I wouldn't have been able to recognize my mom. Past that, things looked a little blurry, as if someone had smeared Vaseline on my glasses."

Melanie walked into the waiting room. Her eyes were watering badly, but she felt elated. "There was no discomfort. No pain at all. And my vision from about three feet away was great—much better than I had ever had. It was really amazing."

RECOVERY
AFTER LASIK

Melanie had a textbook recovery from her Lasik treatment. After the treatment was completed, the technician put in antibiotic and steroid eyedrops. Melanie was given Tylenol with codeine to take later, if necessary, but never needed it. Her eyes were watering and stinging after the procedure, and she wanted to go home to rest in a dimly lit place. A few hours later, she felt well and went out to dinner. She could see clearly for a distance of about three feet and was able to read the menu without a problem. Everything beyond that was slightly blurry. By the time Melanie had finished dinner, her eyes felt slightly gritty, as if she had some dust in them. She went home, took an aspirin, and slept through the night.

The next morning, she woke up and looked straight at the ceiling. It was in sharp focus. "I remember thinking what a miracle it was that I could already see that well." The grittiness that had bothered Melanie the night before had already dissipated, and her biggest complaint was that her eyes periodically felt dry, a sensation that lasted for about a week.

After seeing the doctor, who told her that her eyes were healing nicely, she spent the day visiting museums and that night went to a movie. She could see the screen without glasses and had no problems with halos, glare, or light sensitivity. The following morning, Melanie noticed her vision was significantly sharper than the day before.

Two days after her Lasik procedure, she was back at work and had no problems reading, driving, or using the computer. By the end of the week, she stopped using the eyedrops, as she had been instructed. Her vision was so crisp by that point that she didn't even notice the subtle improvements in her eyesight that gradually occurred over the next month.

Today, Melanie has 20/25 vision. She has noticed that it takes a few moments for her eyes to adjust when she walks from her brightly lit office into the underground parking garage. "My vision is better than it ever was, and life is so much easier now without having to fuss with glasses and contacts."

Diane, a forty-five-year-old physician's assistant, was severely nearsighted. Immediately after the procedure, she looked out the clinic window at the cityscape in the distance. "I could see distances I never could see with glasses, and I started crying. I couldn't believe it. It was a moving experience."

When the anesthetic wore off, Diane felt like she was having a bad contact lens day. Her eyes were burning, red, and gritty. She was also light sensitive. She felt discomfort, not pain, although it periodically hurt to blink. She took some Tylenol with codeine the night after her treatment and used some Advil the following day, but the discomfort disappeared quickly—within twelve hours.

Two days after the treatment, Diane's vision was 20/40, and she was driving without glasses. Her close-up vision, however, lagged behind her ability to see distances. For about six to eight weeks, she had a hard time finding a focal distance for reading. She bought two pairs of reading glasses at the drugstore—one with a weak prescription, the other somewhat stronger—and occasionally used a lighted magnifying glass to read the newspaper. It was frustrating, but two months later, she needed glasses only when reading small print, and the halos she had been seeing around lights at night had completely disappeared.

Ted's recovery from Lasik was similar to Diane's. Before the surgery, the forty-eight-year-old teacher had severe nearsightedness and astigmatism. Immediately after the corneal flap was returned to its place, he could see faces and read large print. That evening, he felt like he had an ill-fitting contact lens in his eye. He wasn't in pain, but he was uncomfortable. He also was light sensitive and saw halos. The next day, he could see distances, but things weren't in sharp focus. "It was like having glasses or contacts and needing a prescription change. Things weren't crisp," he said. He was also having trouble reading, a problem that cleared up about two weeks later. The halos around lights disappeared four months later. These days, he doesn't use glasses at all. "I think it's tremendous."

||||||||||||||||||||||||||||||

RECOVERY
AFTER PRK

No healing process takes place instantaneously, and healing after PRK or Lasik is no exception. For PRK patients, the initial healing phase lasts about a week. Bruce's recovery after PRK was fairly typical. Immediately after the procedure, he received applications of two kinds of eyedrops: steroid drops to control healing and antibiotic drops to prevent infection. The drops needed to be used at regular intervals. He was also given pain pills and anesthetic eyedrops to use as needed. Bruce went home after the treatment and ate dinner. A few hours later, the anesthetic wore off, and he felt like he had a hair in his eye. It was uncomfortable but not bad enough to warrant painkillers. He watched TV and then went to sleep.

The next morning, Bruce went back to see the surgeon. The ride to the office was difficult. Bruce's eye was tearing and was light sensitive. So Bruce put a drop of the anesthetic solution into his eye; the tearing and light sensitivity were greatly diminished.

For the next three days, Bruce felt a mild scratchy sensation in his eye, and his eye watered. Bruce used the anesthetic eyedrops a few times a day, but didn't feel a need for the pain pills. Five days after the PRK treatment, the doctor removed Bruce's protective contact lens. Immediately, Bruce noticed a big improvement in his vision. His eye was still a bit watery, but Bruce was very excited by his improved vision. The next morning, Bruce woke up with no pain, no tearing, and very good vision. "It was golden," he said. He played a game of catch with his son that morning and returned to work the next day. His computer screen looked fuzzy around the edges, but within a few days, it was crisp. For several weeks he noticed slight fluctuations in his vision. "Sometimes my vision was incredibly clear, and sometimes not, as if there were a film over my eyes. It's not that I couldn't see. It's that I couldn't see as well toward the end of the day and at night."

Today, more than a year after his treatment, Bruce's vision is stable and sharp. The halos and slight fluctuations in his vision cleared up within a few months, and the only lenses he wears are nonprescription sunglasses. "I can see the backs of the baseball jerseys from our seats now," he said. "I can go swimming with my kids. I can wrestle with them. I can snuggle with them. The results of the surgery exceeded my expectations, and I still can't believe it."

There's no way to predict how much discomfort a PRK patient will feel after the procedure or how long it will take for vision to stabilize. Most patients complain of only mild discomfort, including tearing, swelling, light sensitivity, and sometimes a stinging or scratchy sensation. A few PRK patients—about two out of ten— experience more significant pain for a day or two after treatment.

If one eye at a time is treated with PRK, a patient can depend on the uncorrected eye while the other eye is healing, so driving and working can resume within several days. People who have both eyes treated with PRK on the same day may not see well enough to drive or read fine print for the first week.

Claire, the fifty-three-year-old photographer, had a quick and easy recovery from PRK. Her eyes felt gritty when the anesthetic wore off, but there was no real pain. To avoid irritating her eyes, her doctor told her not to wear makeup for seven days following the treatment. Within twenty-four hours, her initial discomfort had disappeared. Before laser treatment, her vision was worse than 20/400 in each eye. Now it's 20/20.

For Ethan, recovering from PRK was more difficult. The thirty-two-year-old actor had 20/800 vision in both eyes. He decided to have his right eye treated first. After surgery, his eye was "painful but not unbearable" for a couple of days. It was watery, light sensitive, and slightly red. For two weeks, his vision was blurry, but he could drive using his untreated eye.

A month and a half later, Ethan had his left eye treated. During the procedure, there was absolutely no discomfort, but a few hours later "there was a burning sensation in my eye." Ethan's ophthalmologist removed the protective contact lens, which he thought might be causing the problem, and put some numbing drops in

Ethan's eye. Ethan had some discomfort for two more days, but it was not severe. A few months after the surgery, Ethan had 20/20 vision in both eyes.

After PRK, patients typically use steroid drops in decreasing amounts for up to four months. The first month they commonly use the medication four times a day. Each month, the dosage is decreased. By the final month, most patients need only one drop a day. The eyedrops are critical, because they affect healing and can be adjusted by the doctor to suit a patient's healing pattern.

Lori, a forty-six-year-old special-events planner, learned the hard way how important it is to use the drops diligently. Before having PRK, she couldn't get out of bed without putting her glasses on. For the first two days after the PRK treatment, her eyes were watery and light sensitive. On her doctor's recommendation, she used anesthetic eyedrops as much as needed. She slept a lot, but felt no pain. Four days after the procedure, she saw well enough to drive herself to work.

Lori was happy with her vision, but as the months wore on, she started having difficulty driving at night. Her right eye was somewhat undercorrected. "That could have partially been my fault," she said. "You have to use the steroid drops every eight hours. It's not the kind of thing I'm diligent about, because I didn't understand why I was supposed to do it. I thought I was doing it to keep my eyes moist. I didn't realize the drops were for keeping the correction." Lori had her right eye re-treated, and now has 20/25 vision.

It usually takes several weeks for very good vision to return after PRK, though small changes—sometimes undetectable to the patient—will continue to occur for many months more. After full stabilization, the results will be permanent. Changes in your vision may still occur after the stabilization period, but these changes probably have nothing to do with PRK and would have occurred even without the treatment.

||||||||||||||||||||||||||||

HOW WELL
WILL YOU SEE?

It is impossible to predict precisely how well any specific person will see after laser vision correction, but most patients will no longer need glasses or contact lenses for distance vision. After the initial treatment, about 98 percent of patients will have 20/40 or better vision without glasses; 20/40 vision is good enough to pass the driver's license vision test without glasses. About 90 percent will have 20/20 or better vision without glasses; 20/20 is considered "perfect" vision.

For patients with mild nearsightedness, farsightedness, or astigmatism, the percentages are even better. Patients with severe focusing errors will have lower percentages of 20/20 or 20/40 vision. The general rule is: A higher percentage of accurate results will be obtained in people who require less treatment.

Even those patients who still use glasses for distance vision after the procedure will see better without glasses and use thinner lenses than they did before. If needed, the results can typically be further improved with a repeat laser procedure. This is discussed in the chapter titled "Re-treatments."

These results are very impressive, but it is impossible to tell you exactly what your results will be. No guarantees can be made about the outcome of laser treatment in any individual case, because each person responds in a slightly different way. If you will be satisfied only with "perfect" 20/20 vision without glasses after laser vision correction, then please do not have the treatment. Although this superb vision is achieved for most people, it may not be the result of your treatment. Avoid any doctor or clinic that promises you a specific result, because that simply is not possible.

The quality of vision after laser treatment may be superior or inferior to vision with contact lenses or glasses. Patients often have less glare than they had with contact lenses, and of course the inconvenience and discomfort

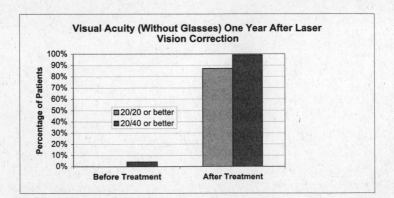

SOURCE: WaveLight Allegretto FDA application

of contact lenses is eliminated. Side vision isn't blocked, as it is with glasses, and there is no longer the problem of dirty, wet, or scratched glasses. However, although excellent vision is almost always obtained with laser vision correction, no promises or guarantees can be made.

‖‖‖‖‖‖‖‖‖‖‖‖‖‖‖‖‖‖‖

THE HEALING RESPONSE:
THE BIG VARIABLE

If eyes were made of marble, we could correct every one of them to a perfect 20/20. But eyes are made of living tissue. As can be expected, not all eyes display the same healing response. The individual healing response, which cannot be predicted precisely, affects the patient's final vision. Your eye's healing response cannot be predicted by how fast other parts of your body heal and cannot be determined by testing.

Fortunately, there is much less variation in the healing pattern of the eye than in many other parts of the body. Most people exhibit a predictable healing pattern. As the eye heals during the first several weeks or months, there is a slight tendency for the eye to revert toward its initial state: nearsighted eyes will regress very mildly back toward nearsightedness and farsighted eyes will regress slightly back toward farsightedness. Doctors take this tendency into account, and will create a small overcorrection initially. As a result, most patients will notice that their vision sharpens during the first several weeks or months of the healing period.

Some patients display a healing pattern known as regression, in which the eyes revert a greater amount than is normal. These people may have excellent vision during the early healing period, which then regresses into an undercorrection. Fortunately, undercorrections are very easily improved with a re-treatment.

Extensive exposure to ultraviolet light, such as from the sun or from tanning salons, during the first six months after treatment may cause some patients to undergo regression. It is very important for patients to protect their eyes from excessive amounts of ultraviolet light by wearing sunglasses when in the sun during the first six months after treatment, though small amounts of sun exposure will not be detrimental. Skiing, high-altitude sports, water sports, golf, and beach going involve a great deal of ultraviolet exposure, so it is particularly important to protect your eyes by wearing sunglasses during these activities. Excessive ultraviolet light is also harmful to other parts of the eye (it can cause cataracts and damage the retina), so it is wise for everyone, whether or not they have recently had laser vision correction, to protect their eyes from the harmful effects of the sun. Think of how the sun ages and damages the skin—it does the same type of damage to the eyes!

Everyone heals differently, and the differences can significantly affect your final result. This is one of the reasons why it is so important to pick your doctor carefully. Regardless of the accuracy of the laser, it is still the doctor who uses the laser and then manages your healing response afterward. Be sure you understand your postoperative instructions, so that you will do everything you can to help with your final result.

||||||||||||||||||||||||||||

COMPLICATIONS:
WHAT CAN GO WRONG?

Laser vision correction is subject to complications, but the complication rate is very low. Patients often ask if one of these complications is likely to occur to them. It is impossible to predict whether a complication will occur in any specific case. Complications are rare but will be more common in people with high amounts of nearsightedness, farsightedness, or astigmatism, because these people require larger amounts of treatment. Most complications can be partially or totally corrected through a repeat laser procedure.

Patients commonly ask if they can go blind from the laser treatment. To the best of our knowledge, no person anywhere has ever gone blind from laser vision correction. A severe infection could result in greatly decreased vision, though probably not blindness. Fortunately, further laser treatment or other surgery could improve vision in almost every situation.

During the first few months of healing, it is common

for patients to experience difficulty with vision, including blurred vision, double vision, increased halos, glare, and light sensitivity. A foreign-body sensation and excess tearing will also occur in many people during the first month of healing. These symptoms are generally temporary and are a normal part of the healing process. Some people will experience difficulties that persist longer than one month.

The most significant problems of laser vision correction include undercorrection and overcorrection, increased optical aberrations in low light, dry eyes, infection, flap problems, ectasia, and decrease in best corrected vision.

UNDERCORRECTION OR OVERCORRECTION

By far the most common complication of laser vision correction is undercorrection or overcorrection. These complications occur because the patient experiences an abnormal healing response or because the laser energy removed slightly too much or too little tissue.

In the case of an undercorrection, the patient will be left with some degree of the initial focusing problem, though much less so than before. Further laser treatment, known as an "enhancement" or a "touch-up," can then be used to further improve the vision.

An overcorrection will result in a reversal of the vision focusing error: an overcorrection of nearsightedness will result in farsightedness, and vice versa. In most cases, an enhancement laser treatment can be performed to improve the resulting focusing error.

Undercorrections and overcorrections are the main

reason that all patients do not have perfect 20/20 vision after laser vision treatment. No patient can be guaranteed perfect vision after laser vision correction. If you will be satisfied only with 20/20 vision, then you should not have the procedure, because this result cannot be guaranteed.

INCREASED OPTICAL ABERRATIONS IN LOW LIGHT

Every person, whether or not they have laser vision correction, has some degree of vision imperfection, especially in low light. These vision irregularities, known as aberrations, are much more prominent in darkness than in bright light. To see this for yourself, look at the moon at night with no other bright lights around, using your glasses or contact lenses. You will notice that the edges of the moon are not crisp. Instead, there is always some degree of halo or glare around the edges of the moon. These vision irregularities are typically much less noticeable when you view the moon during the daytime, when the overall lighting level is higher.

Before civilization, human beings were hunters and gatherers of food, and they worked only in the daytime. Our eyes evolved to see much better in the daylight than in darkness. As a result, we have less optimal vision in darkness, with significant optical aberrations. Many animals are just the opposite: Animals that are nighttime hunters have much better vision in darkness than in bright light.

Optical aberrations in low light are more common in

people with large amounts of optical correction as well as those who have particularly large pupils in the dark.

Newer lasers with larger treatment patterns have dramatically lessened the problem of optical aberrations after laser vision correction. Many people notice some temporarily increased glare or halos for the first several weeks after laser vision correction. Typically, this is something that is noticed, but is not particularly bothersome. For most people, the degree of halo and glare returns to pretreatment levels or even better by about three months.

For several weeks after having PRK, Bruce saw starbursts or halos around stoplights when he drove home at night. "It happens less and less," he said. "When it's pitch-black and there's only one light, that's when I get the starburst."

If increased optical aberrations remain after six months and are bothersome, they can usually be treated with a wavefront-guided enhancement.

DRY EYES

Many people experience increased dryness of the eyes during the first few days or weeks of the healing period after laser vision correction. For most people, the feeling of dryness and irritation is merely a minor inconvenience and is treated by using moisturizing eyedrops.

Dryness is more common in patients who have dry eyes before laser vision correction or who live in very dry environments. It is more troublesome during the winter months, when the humidity is lower. Dryness will cause irritation of the eyes and may cause a temporary mild decrease in the sharpness of the vision.

Melanie's dryness after Lasik was fairly typical: "My eyes felt a little scratchy for about a week. Nothing drastic, just something I noticed. It felt better when I put in the wetting drops. But after a week or so, I found that I didn't need the wetting drops anymore." Some people experience more significant dryness after laser vision correction, which in very rare cases can last for many months.

If you are bothered by dryness after laser vision correction, you will need to use moisturizing drops. Air blowing across the face will dry out the eyes, so avoid wind, air conditioners, or open car windows. Omega-3 pills or liquid, which can be bought without a prescription in the drugstore or health food store, are very effective when ingested daily in treating dryness of the eyes. Often a humidifier in the bedroom or thicker drops at bedtime will also be useful. In the rare case of prolonged dryness, special anti-inflammatory drops are usually very effective.

INFECTION

Just as with surgery on any part of the body, the eye is susceptible to infection during the early healing period after laser vision correction. You will be asked to follow certain instructions, including using antibiotic eyedrops and keeping water and makeup away from the eyes, during the first few days after your procedure. Carefully following these instructions will decrease the infection rate to much less than 1 percent. Even if an infection were to occur, use of antibiotic eyedrops should control the infection.

FLAP PROBLEMS

Creation of the protective corneal flap is the part of the Lasik procedure that most worries patients. In fact, in the hands of a skilled and experienced surgeon, flap problems occur less than 1 percent of the time and are usually minor in nature. The main flap problem is sliding and wrinkling of the flap, which most commonly occurs during the first day after the procedure, before the flap has healed solidly in place. This can occur by accidentally touching the flap with your finger or medicine dropper, or if the eye becomes overly dry during the first night. Movement of the flap will blur the vision, so your doctor will need to adjust the flap, which is painless and requires just a few minutes.

In very rare situations, the flap creation will not be optimal. When this occurs, the doctor will usually not proceed with the laser portion of the treatment. Instead, the doctor will ask you to wait several months for the flap to heal firmly and will then perform the laser treatment.

ECTASIA

Ectasia (also known as keractectasia) is the condition in which the rigidity of the cornea is not adequate. In patients with ectasia, the shape of the cornea, and the vision, change over time. Laser treatment cannot be used to improve the vision, because removal of corneal tissue would only further weaken the cornea.

Ectasia is present in around one in 2,500 people in the general population. These people should not have Lasik, because it may cause the condition to advance at a faster rate.

Most people with ectasia develop the condition in their teenage years, but some will develop the condition later in life. Doctors use many tests to attempt to determine if a person has ectasia or is likely to develop ectasia in the future. Unfortunately, these tests do not identify all of the people at risk for ectasia. There are rare people who will test normally but who are genetically programmed to develop ectasia. If such a person has laser vision correction, particularly the Lasik variation, the ectasia may become evident shortly after the laser treatment, earlier than it would otherwise appear.

Because of the flap, Lasik affects more of the fibers in the cornea than PRK. If there is concern that a person is at a more significant risk for ectasia, then PRK is a safer alternative than Lasik.

The treatment for ectasia is to wear glasses or contact lenses. In more advanced cases, contact lenses are preferable. In extreme cases, the weak cornea is surgically replaced with a new cornea. A new treatment using vitamin B2 eyedrops and ultraviolet light is very promising.

Decrease in Best Corrected Vision

Best corrected vision is the best vision obtainable when wearing the optimal pair of glasses or contact lenses. It is a measure of the best vision possible with glasses or contacts. Of course, you probably will no longer use glasses or contact lenses for distance vision after the surgery, so you may not even be aware if your best possible vision is slightly different.

For the majority of people, a mild decrease in best corrected vision is usually not noticed. A moderate loss of best corrected visual acuity would be noticed by every patient and might make it hard to work in occupations that require fine vision. Severe loss of best corrected visual acuity is exceedingly rare and in fact has not occurred in any of the FDA-sponsored tests.

Some professionals, such as commercial airplane pilots, care very much about their best corrected vision. These pilots must have best corrected vision of 20/20 in both eyes to maintain their licenses, so they should carefully consider the small risk of less than 20/20 best corrected vision.

Commonly, best corrected vision actually improves after laser vision correction, particularly with wavefront custom laser treatment. Patients after treatment will often have 20/15 vision, whereas prior to laser treatment their vision with the perfect glasses or contact lenses was 20/20.

||||||||||||||||||||||||||||||||

RE-TREATMENTS

Not all patients get a satisfactory result from laser treatment. This may be due to undercorrection, overcorrection, or one of the complications described previously. By far the most common problem with eye laser treatment is an undercorrection or overcorrection.

Patients who experience undercorrection or overcorrection can usually undergo a second procedure, known as an enhancement, to obtain a better correction. In most cases, a significant improvement in the vision will occur, but it is important to realize that this, too, is a laser procedure and therefore has similar risks as the first laser procedure. It is possible but rare that your vision can be worse after an enhancement procedure. Complications can occur, even if no complications occurred during your first procedure.

If your vision is quite good after your laser treatment, but not perfect, you should consider carefully whether you want to have an enhancement procedure. Maybe you can easily adapt by wearing glasses on a limited basis, such as for driving or watching movies. If your vision is really not satisfactory, then an enhancement procedure is a good idea.

Overall, around 10 percent of patients undergo enhancement procedures, though your likelihood will vary significantly depending on your degree of nearsightedness, farsightedness, and astigmatism. Over 25 percent of patients with extremely high degrees of nearsightedness, farsightedness, and astigmatism are likely to require enhancement procedures.

Lori ended up slightly undercorrected in both eyes after having PRK, which meant she was still somewhat nearsighted. She had excellent vision for close-up work, but distances were a problem—especially when driving at night. She got prescription glasses as a "security blanket," she said, "because it's a little scary to wait until you get right up to the street signs" to read them. She decided to have an enhancement procedure on her right eye.

The enhancement, Lori said, "was a snap, because I knew what was going to happen. It was like seeing a movie the second time." The procedure was identical to Lori's first surgery, except it took even less time to complete. She took a pain pill for less than twenty-four hours and never experienced any pain, swelling, or light sensitivity. "Having one eye done was a breeze, because I could rely on the other eye. It was like it didn't happen," she said. Within three days, she was driving without glasses, wearing makeup, and was back at work.

Ted decided to have touch-up surgery four months after he first had Lasik. He was 20/40 in one eye and

20/70 in the other, and was straining to see distances when driving.

The touch-up Lasik procedure differed slightly from the first operation. Rather than making a new flap in the cornea, the doctor was able to see the outline of the original flap and reopen it using a small instrument. The procedure itself was painless, but Ted experienced slightly more postoperative discomfort after the second surgery than he had felt after the first. The corneal flap irritated his eyelid. "It felt like something was in my eye, and I wanted to rub it," he says. The doctor put in a protective contact lens, and the pain disappeared.

The next day, Ted could read license plates. His vision had improved to 20/25, and he wasn't feeling any discomfort. Today, he doesn't need glasses for reading or distance.

||||||||||||||||||||||||||||

ONE EYE OR TWO?

As a patient you must decide: Do you want both eyes treated on the same day, or each eye on a separate day? Each approach has advantages and disadvantages. Your decision may also depend on whether you are having Lasik or PRK.

If both eyes are treated on the same day, then the healing for both eyes will occur at the same time. You will not have to go through two separate healing periods. However, your vision will be limited in both eyes at the same time as they simultaneously heal.

Lasik patients usually experience a rapid return of vision, so most Lasik patients elect to have both eyes treated on the same day. Most, but not all, Lasik patients who have both eyes treated on the same day are able to drive and return to work the very next day.

After having a conversation with his doctor, David decided to have Lasik on both eyes on the same day. He knew that it might take longer for him to be able to see clearly and return to his normal life, but he couldn't tolerate contact lenses and didn't want to have to wear his thick glasses lens on one eye and nothing on the other while recovering from the Lasik. "The perceived benefit to me seemed so much greater than the risk," he said. For two days after his surgery, David had difficulty seeing, but by the third day, he was in good shape. In his mind, the temporary inconvenience was worthwhile.

PRK patients typically experience five or six days during the initial healing period with some limitation of their activities. Although the vision will be fine for most activities, it may be difficult for some people to drive or to read extensively. This varies significantly from person to person; many are able to drive and work at a computer during the first week, but others are not. For a few additional weeks, most PRK patients will see well enough for the majority of work activities, including reading, but not for extremely fine visual tasks.

The majority of PRK patients choose to have both eyes treated on the same day. This is probably the easiest way if you are able to take five to seven days off from most reading and driving activities.

Some Lasik and PRK patients choose to have the eyes treated on separate days. Treating one eye at a time is usually less convenient, but some patients feel greater confidence this way. When one eye is treated at a time, you can typically resume most activities the next day, because you can see well out of the untreated eye with a contact lens or glasses while the treated eye is healing.

Ethan had his eyes treated on different days. After the first PRK procedure, his vision out of the treated eye was blurry. While the treated eye was healing, he wore his corrective contact lens in the untreated eye. He could drive, read, and go to work. "I would just concentrate on seeing out of the one eye," he said. "It's difficult, but you can do it."

Nicole, a thirty-seven-year-old actress, also had PRK performed on her eyes on separate occasions. After her first treatment, her eye was tearing and scratchy. She used anesthetic eyedrops to dull the discomfort and slept a lot during the first two days. For the first month or two after the procedure, Nicole wore her corrective contact lens in the untreated eye. Her naturally dry eyes, however, caused the eye with the contact lens to become red and gritty. After a few weeks, Nicole decided to leave the lens out. "I just relied on my one treated eye until the second eye was treated," she said. "That was fine."

Nicole's second procedure was easy in comparison to the first. She experienced less discomfort afterward and felt like "more of an old pro," she explained. "For the first few days, I covered the newly treated eye and read with my one good eye."

||||||||||||||||||||||||||

HOW TO
CHOOSE A DOCTOR

If you think surgical correction of nearsightedness, far-sightedness, and/or astigmatism may be for you, the most important choice you will make is the doctor. A conscientious surgeon will help you decide whether laser treatment is right for you by highlighting the pros and cons as they relate to your particular situation. The surgeon should discuss the advantages and disadvantages of PRK, Lasik, and nonlaser procedures to help you choose which technique is best for you. The surgeon will also perform the procedure.

The role of the doctor cannot be overemphasized. Some clinics would like you to think that the laser does all the work and that the surgeon is not very important. Nothing could be further from the truth. Remember—the laser is the tool the surgeon uses to correct your vision and, like other tools, the way it is used makes all the difference. The laser does not decide what to do—the doctor does. The laser performs the task that it is programmed for, so the measurements and information given to the laser by the doctor are critical. Also, the laser will not be monitoring your progress or initiating adjustments after the procedure—the doctor will.

The surgeon will decide which equipment to use and will make sure that the equipment is properly maintained and calibrated.

Be wary of clinics that de-emphasize the surgeon, and make sure that you know your surgeon and feel comfortable with his or her manner, education, and experience. Select a doctor that you trust and who you think has good judgment.

Be wary also of slick advertisements. A good advertisement means nothing more than the clinic has a good advertising agency. It does not mean that the doctor is right for you.

Be careful about referrals from other eye doctors. Many eye doctors have financial arrangements with specific laser clinics or surgeons and the referring doctor will receive financial benefit if the procedure is performed by the suggested clinic or surgeon. Carefully question the referring eye doctor and the laser surgeon to be sure that you know the details of this financial arrangement and make sure that you feel confident with your choice.

Carefully check the credentials of the surgeon. See if the doctor is board certified in ophthalmology and make sure that you respect the doctor's education, training, and experience. Has the doctor just started performing surgery to treat nearsightedness, farsightedness, and astigmatism, or has the doctor been doing so for many years? How many Lasik or PRK procedures has the doctor performed and how many does he or she perform each week? Is Lasik and PRK a major part of the doctor's practice or just one of many parts? As a consumer, you need to be aware that there are very significant quality differences among surgeons and among laser centers, and that these quality differences may have an impact upon your chances of complication and your final visual result.

Does the doctor listen to you, and does the doctor clearly answer all your questions? Does the doctor seem to care about you and your individual needs?

|||||||||||||||||||||||||||||||

IF YOU ARE
OVER THIRTY-FIVE

If you are over thirty-five years old, please read this section very carefully. It may seem confusing at first, but it is very important that you understand it.

As people approach forty to forty-five, they begin to lose the ability to change their visual focus from far to near. When their eyes are adjusted for distance, either with glasses, contact lenses, or with laser eye treatment, there is difficulty in seeing clearly up close.

If you don't wear glasses or contact lenses, you will begin to need glasses for clear close vision when you approach forty to forty-five years of age. These reading glasses are often called "magnifying glasses." If you need glasses or contact lenses for clear distance vision, you will need to wear a separate, additional pair of glasses for reading, or use a combination of distance and near glasses known as bifocal, trifocal, blended, or progressive glasses. Alternatively, you will need to take off your distance glasses or contact lenses in order to see clearly up close, because you will be unable to see near objects clearly with your distance glasses on.

People commonly refer to this condition as "farsightedness," but, in fact, it is not true farsightedness at all. True farsightedness (hyperopia) is an inherent lack of focusing power in the eye and is not caused by getting older. The medical term for the change that occurs with aging is "presbyopia," which comes from the Greek words meaning "old vision." (Unfortunately, there is no English word for this condition other than the awkward "presbyopia.") Everybody develops presbyopia.

If you are nearsighted, farsighted, or have astigmatism and are developing presbyopia, you will probably need bifocal or trifocal glasses. The upper lenses of the bifocals are for distance vision; the lower are for close-up vision. Some people prefer trifocals, in which there are three pairs of lenses—an upper pair for distance, a middle pair for middle distances (about three to six feet), and a bottom pair for objects one to three feet away. Blended or progressive lenses also have distance vision on the top and near vision at the bottom.

Bifocal contact lenses are available but generally do not provide sharp vision for both distance and near.

For those of you approaching or in this age group, you and your doctor must decide how best to correct your vision when you develop presbyopia. This decision must be made regardless of how you choose to correct your refractive error—either surgically or with glasses or contact lenses. People who have already begun to use bifocals, trifocals, or reading glasses understand this, but people who have not yet crossed this threshold or who simply remove their glasses when they read usually find this confusing.

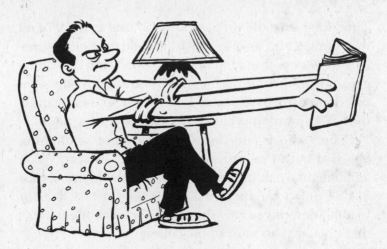

"Honey, I think my arms are getting too short!"

You have three choices regarding your presbyopia. None of these options cure the presbyopia, so no option is ideal. Each has pros and cons. The key is to select the option that is most suitable for you.

1. *Adjust for distance.* Both eyes can be fully adjusted for clear distance vision. The patient will need to wear reading glasses ("magnifying glasses") for good close vision, usually beginning sometime between the ages of forty and fifty. This might be referred to as the "normal" situation, because most people start to need reading glasses at about that age.

Nicole, who was thirty-seven, decided to have both eyes adjusted for distance. Four years later, at the age of forty-one, she started noticing subtle differences in her close-up vision. "It's not that I can't see up close," she explained, "but it's not as crystal sharp as it used to be.

Threading a needle isn't as easy as it used to be. When I was younger and wore contacts, I would take off my contact lenses to thread needles. I don't need reading glasses yet, but the perfect precision of close-up sight that I used to have when I was younger is not quite there. I know it's just basically a part of getting older."

Claire, who is fifty-three, echoes those sentiments. She had both eyes corrected for clear distance vision and bought a pair of reading glasses at the pharmacy for $14. "I only wear them if I'm reading in bad light or reading tiny, tiny print," she said. "For someone my age, that's better than most of my colleagues."

2. *Monovision.* Monovision is when one eye is adjusted for distance vision and one eye for near vision. Monovision is often created with contact lenses for people over forty years old and can be replicated with laser vision correction. In monovision, one eye is primarily used at a time for ideal focus. The "distance" eye is primarily used to see far-off objects. The "close-up" eye is primarily used to see near objects. Both eyes are used all the time, but one is generally primary, depending on the distance of the viewed object. Peripheral vision is unaffected and depth perception is usually only mildly affected.

The main advantage of monovision is that patients often will not have to use glasses for distance vision or for near vision. The main disadvantage is that the patient is subconsciously relying on one eye at a time, and some people do not like this. Monovision will dramatically decrease the need for glasses, but may not free you from glasses completely. Some people with monovision will still use glasses in particular situations where they require excellent vision out of both eyes. Some, but not all, monovision patients will use glasses when driving a car (especially at night) or doing extensive reading. Other monovision patients will almost never use glasses.

Monovision is achieved by purposefully leaving one eye somewhat nearsighted, either with contact lenses or when having laser treatment. Usually, this is the non-dominant eye (often but not always the left eye in a right-handed person or the right eye in a left-handed person). If a patient chooses monovision and for some reason does not like it afterward, the "near" eye can usually be corrected for distance in a second laser procedure. This will eliminate the remaining nearsightedness.

A person with both eyes corrected for distance can, if he or she prefers, typically go back at a later date and have one eye readjusted for monovision. Getting completely used to monovision generally takes several weeks but may take several months, because you are breaking very well-established ways of using your eyes. People rarely ask to have monovision eliminated after they get adjusted to it.

Paul, a forty-three-year-old doctor, decided to have laser vision correction performed on his right eye. He improved his vision in that eye from 20/200 to 20/20, but he left his other eye uncorrected. He opted for monovision, he said, because "I'd like to be able to read without glasses. I'm also a microsurgeon. I like to be able to hold things very close to see them. If I had both eyes adjusted for distance, I'd lose that ability very soon."

It took Paul about three weeks to mentally and physically adjust to monovision. Initially, he saw subtle halos in the dark, and his reading vision in the corrected eye was poor. He continued to wear a contact lens in his untreated eye for distance and didn't operate for three weeks after the surgery. Now, more than a year after his procedure, Paul doesn't require corrective lenses for any task. When reading and operating, he relies on his nearsighted eye. When he's driving or at the movies, his distance eye takes over.

3. *Mild monovision.* This is a compromise between full distance vision in each eye and full monovision. In mild monovision, one eye is left with only a small amount of nearsightedness. This will cause only a small decrease in distance vision in that eye, but will aid somewhat in midrange and close-up vision. For many patients forty-five or older, this mild monovision is a reasonable solution to the problem of nearsightedness, farsightedness, and astigmatism combined with the aging changes of loss of focusing. The degree of mild monovision is adjustable, based on the patient's age and visual demands.

How can you determine if monovision or mild monovision might be right for you? During your consultation, your doctor can easily show you monovision with test glasses or contact lenses. Most people will determine whether they like monovision or not within just a few minutes of testing in the doctor's office. If you desire, you can have a special pair of monovision glasses or contact lenses made in order to test for a longer period of time at home or work.

Lori decided that, at the age of forty-six, mild monovision made more sense than a full correction for distance. After having laser vision correction, her vision improved to 20/25 in the right eye and 20/40 in the left. She doesn't need corrective lenses for reading or distance. "The joke among my friends is that I'm now the only one who doesn't need glasses," she said. "I love it."

There are only a few times during the day that Lori notices she has monovision—when she's putting on makeup or reading for long periods of time. When she looks up from a book, it takes a few seconds for her eyes to readjust to see distances. And, she added, "When you're putting makeup on, if you close the eye that's corrected for close-up work, you're left with an eye that has distance vision and doesn't see as well up close. Other than that, you never notice."

Lori is thrilled with the results of her monovision. "It's freed me to see," she remarked. "I don't have to think about seeing, whereas when you wear glasses, you always think about seeing. You wake up in the middle of the night, and you can't go to the bathroom without a pair of glasses on. Now I go past the mirror in the middle of the night, and I'm startled because I think someone's in the room with me. Then I realize it's me. I've just never been able to see that far."

A small number of people over forty with nearsightedness do not wear bifocal, trifocal, or progressive glasses, but merely take off their distance glasses when they want to read close-up. The key question you must ask yourself is: Can you read up close with your distance glasses on? If you *must* take off your distance glasses to read up close, then you have presbyopia. People with presbyopia who get both eyes fully corrected for distance vision will then need to use reading glasses to see clearly close-up. If you currently simply take off your glasses to read up close, then you should carefully consider whether or not you really want to have laser treatment to eliminate completely your distance glasses prescription.

|||||||||||||||||||||||||||||

THE MOST
COMMONLY ASKED QUESTIONS
ABOUT LASER VISION
CORRECTION

What are the odds of eliminating my need for distance glasses with laser treatment?

Overall, 80 percent of people after treatment will have perfect (20/20 or better) vision without using glasses or contact lenses, and 98 percent of patients will see well enough without glasses or contacts to pass the driver's license vision test (20/40 or better). More accurate results are achieved when using the newer wavefront technology. If the vision after the initial treatment is not as ideal as desired, a second treatment (known as an enhancement) can typically be performed.

Does laser vision correction hurt?

There is only mild discomfort during the procedure, usually less than having your teeth cleaned. For the first few days after Lasik, there is usually a mild scratchy sensation. PRK patients will experience a little longer and greater discomfort than Lasik patients.

Can I go blind from laser vision correction?

Although this is theoretically possible, to the best of our knowledge it has never happened. The most serious risk of vision loss is an infection, so it is important to use antibiotic eyedrops and to follow your doctor's instructions after the procedure. Even in this exceedingly remote possibility, the vision could usually be restored by a repeat laser procedure or by other surgery, such as a corneal transplant.

What about the long-term results? Will my eyes deteriorate in the future?

Since 1988, tens of millions of Lasik and PRK procedures have been performed around the world and many careful studies have been performed. There is no evidence of any adverse long-term effects on the health of the eye. The making of a flap, a major part of the Lasik procedure, has been used since the 1970s without negative long-term effects.

Which technique is better for me: Lasik or PRK?

Most doctors recommend Lasik over PRK, except in specific situations, due to the more rapid healing. However, in your particular situation, PRK may be more appropriate. Most patients can have their treatment using either Lasik or PRK. In some cases, one eye is treated with Lasik and the other eye with PRK. It is important to carefully consider the pros and cons of each technique.

What about other techniques to permanently correct nearsightedness, farsightedness, and astigmatism?

Several nonlaser techniques are available. Permanent, plastic lenses, known as lens implants, can be placed inside the eye. Lens implants may be combined with the removal of the natural crystalline lens from the eye. Conductive keratoplasty (CK) uses radio frequency energy to correct farsightedness. Although laser treatment is preferable to these other techniques in most situations, a nonlaser method will be more appropriate in some specific cases.

Will I need to wear an eye patch after the procedure?
No, though some people will need to wear a special contact lens for a few days.

I've heard that ultraviolet light can cause cancer. Can this laser cause cancer?
There is no risk of cancer from Lasik or PRK.

Will I be able to see anything during the procedure?
Yes. During the procedure, you will be asked to look at a blinking light. This will help to maintain proper alignment of the eye during the procedure. However, you will not be able to see any details of the treatment.

What if I move during the procedure?
Patients worry about this a great deal, and their fear is unnecessary. Eyes move naturally all the time, so the laser has a built-in eye tracker which follows the eyes as they move. Also, the doctor can immediately stop the procedure at any time and resume when the patient is ready.

What if I blink during the procedure?
Your eye will be held open by a device known as a speculum, which usually doesn't hurt. You will not be able to blink.

Will laser vision correction cause cataracts or influence the later treatment of cataracts?

Laser vision correction is not known to cause cataracts and does not affect the removal of cataracts. However, if you know you will need cataract surgery in the near future, there is no need to undergo laser vision correction; your nearsightedness, farsightedness, or astigmatism can be corrected as a part of the cataract implant surgery.

Will there be any limitations on my activities after laser treatment?

There are no limitations on your activities, except that you will be asked to avoid getting water into your eye and wearing eye makeup during the first several days. Of course, you should not resume activities such as driving until your vision is adequate.

If I don't get a perfect 20/20 correction, will I be able to wear contacts after laser treatment?

Very rarely, a patient will not get a full correction with laser vision correction and will want to wear contact lenses. The general rule is: If you could wear contact lenses before the procedure, then you should be able to wear them afterward. If you were unable to wear contacts before the procedure, then you probably will not be able to wear them afterward. There are some exceptions to this rule. After laser vision correction the cornea has a slightly different shape, so some patients who could wear contacts before the procedure will not find an adequate fit after. However, because there are so many contacts now available, this would be exceedingly rare. More often, the opposite is true: Some patients who could not tolerate the thick lenses that were necessary before the laser procedure can wear thin contacts after the procedure.

If I don't get a perfect 20/20 correction, will I be able to have a repeat procedure to improve the results?

In most but not all cases a "touch-up" or "enhancement" procedure can be performed to improve the vision, usually to 20/20.

My distance vision has recently been getting worse. Will laser eye surgery stop the eyes from getting worse?

No. Laser vision correction can correct nearsightedness, farsightedness, and astigmatism that is currently present, but cannot stop these naturally occurring conditions from developing in the future. If your distance vision is significantly changing, you may want to delay the procedure until your distance vision stabilizes. In most people, distance vision stabilizes during the late teen years or early twenties, though significant changes can occur at other times.

What are the most common negative side effects of laser vision treatment?

Undercorrection or overcorrection are the most common negative results of laser vision correction. Usually this can be corrected with a second, "touch-up" procedure. Increased glare or halos in low light are common during the healing period but almost always resolve over time. Many people have dryness in the eyes for several weeks, or even months, after the treatment, which is treated with drops or pills.

I am very nervous about the procedure. Is this normal?
Can I take Valium before the procedure?

Everyone is nervous about having a treatment performed on his or her eyes. This is normal human nature. Most doctors will give relaxation medication prior to the procedure, but it is important to take only medication prescribed by your doctor.

PART
II

||||||||||||||||||||||||||||||||

ADDITIONAL
INFORMATION
—
FOR THOSE
WHO WANT TO KNOW
MORE

||||||||||||||||||||||||||

WHAT
DOES "20/20" MEAN?

The most important aspect of vision is known as "acuity," the ability of the eye to distinguish fine details. Acuity is measured by the smallest letters the patient can see on an eye chart. In the United States, we use twenty feet as a standard testing distance, and so "20" is always used as the first number in the visual-acuity measurement.

The second number in the measurement refers to the size of the smallest letters the patient can see. Size 20 letters are the smallest letters that most people with "perfect" vision can see at the standard twenty-foot testing distance. Size 40 letters are twice as big, and size 200 letters are ten times as big. Thus, a patient with 20/40 vision, when tested at 20 feet, can see down to the size 40 letters, but cannot see letters smaller than that.

Each eye is measured separately and has its own distance acuity. There are actually three different measurements of distance acuity for each eye: visual acuity without glasses or contact lenses (known as "uncorrected" vision), visual acuity with the current glasses or contacts (which may not be very accurate!), and visual acuity with the perfect glasses or contact lenses (also known as "best corrected visual acuity"). So a nearsighted person might have 20/200 vision without glasses, 20/30 vision with the current glasses, and 20/20 vision with the best possible glasses.

Normally we consider 20/20 to be "perfect" vision, although a small percentage of people (about 10 percent) have even better vision—20/15. People with 20/25 or 20/30 uncorrected vision have very good, but not perfect, distance vision. Although their friends may be able to read smaller letters than they can at a distance, these people will probably get by fine without glasses for dis-

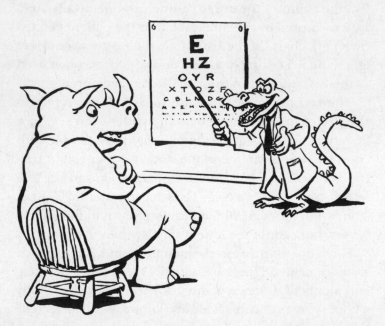

tance vision or may use glasses on a very limited basis, such as for driving or watching movies.

Most people with 20/40 or 20/50 uncorrected vision use glasses for some things but not for everything. He or she will wear glasses to drive but might not wear glasses around the house and will probably feel comfortable swimming or playing most sports without glasses. However, this is highly individual; some people with this vision will wear glasses almost all the time. In most states, a person must see at least 20/40 to pass the driver's license vision test. People with uncorrected vision worse than 20/40 legally have to wear corrective lenses to drive. Most people with uncorrected vision worse than 20/50 will use glasses for distance vision most of the time. However, people vary in this regard; some prefer blurry vision to wearing corrective lenses.

Do all people with uncorrected 20/20 acuity have the same vision? No, other aspects of vision are also important. Dim lighting, side lighting, and glare can affect some people's vision more than others. This is known as contrast sensitivity. Contrast sensitivity can be measured, but this test is time-consuming to perform and has not gained widespread popularity.

HOW TO READ A GLASSES PRESCRIPTION

+2.00 – 1.25 @ 90. This is a glasses prescription for a patient with farsightedness and astigmatism.

The first number (+2.00) is the amount of nearsightedness or farsightedness (a minus sign is for nearsightedness; a plus sign is for farsightedness). The second number (–1.25) is the amount of astigmatism, while the third number (@ 90) is the direction (axis) of the astigmatism. If there is no astigmatism, the prescription will have only one number, in this example +2.00.

Glasses prescriptions are in diopters, which measure how strongly the lenses bend the light rays. This should not be confused with visual acuity measurements! For example, a 2.00 lens does not mean that the eye sees 20/200; however, the higher the diopter number of your glasses, the worse your uncorrected visual acuity will be.

HOW TO READ A CONTACT LENS PRESCRIPTION

+1.75 – 1.25 @ 90 / 8.6 / 13.8

Your contact lens prescription will be slightly different from your glasses prescription. The first set of numbers will be the nearsightedness or farsightedness and astigmatism, but these numbers will vary slightly from your glasses prescription. Also, the contact lens prescription will include the curvature, diameter, manufacturer, and model of the contact lens. In the above example, 8.6 refers to the curvature of the lens and 13.8 is the diameter.

||||||||||||||||||||||||||||

WHAT IS A LASER?
WHAT IS AN
EXCIMER LASER?

A laser is a machine that produces a special type of light that can be very accurately focused. Unlike the light produced by ordinary lightbulbs, laser light is both uniform and coherent. "Uniform" means that each light ray is always one precise wavelength (energy), whereas ordinary light is a mixture of many different wavelengths. "Coherent" means that the light rays are highly synchronized in space and time. Because of these qualities, laser light can be very intense and can be focused very precisely, making laser light useful in medicine and industry.

Different lasers produce light of different wavelengths. Some lasers produce light that is visible to the human eye, whereas other lasers produce light that is invisible, such as ultraviolet or infrared light.

The term "laser" is short for "Light Amplification by Stimulated Emission of Radiation," the process by which a laser produces its light. Some people become alarmed when they hear the word "radiation," because they know that some types of radiation (such as X-rays) can cause cancer. All types of light, including the normal light that we see, are a form of radiation. You do not have to be concerned: Eye lasers use light, but these lasers do not cause cancer.

The excimer laser used in laser vision correction uses argon and fluorine gases to produce a beam of invisible, ultraviolet light. The laser light is then focused by a series of lenses, bounced off a series of mirrors, and mixed to create a more even beam pattern. Excimer lasers are very complex devices that can cost hundreds of thousands of dollars. In spite of the cost, excimer lasers have found a wide variety of uses in industry, ranging from glass etching to the sterilization of wines. The excimer laser can precisely remove tissue without causing scarring, which makes it ideal for reshaping the cornea.

Albert Einstein first proposed the principle behind

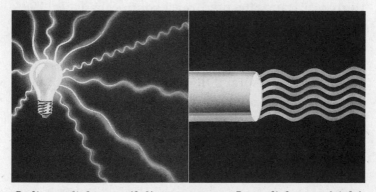

Ordinary light rays (left) are uneven. Laser light rays (right) are highly synchronized in space and time, and are one precise wavelength.

the laser in 1916, but it was not until 1960 that the first laser was built.

While most people are unaware of it, lasers are almost everywhere. Compact disc players use a laser beam to read the information encoded on the compact disc (which can be music, movies, or computer data). Lasers are also used extensively in communications, the military, and manufacturing, as well as in science. For example, a laser beam has been bounced off the moon and has measured the distance from the earth to the moon to within one inch.

Lasers are used in many fields of medicine, and their uses are increasing. Lasers can be used to remove wrinkles from the skin as well as polyps from the vocal cords. Orthopedic surgeons use lasers to remove tissue from inside damaged joints, and neurosurgeons use them to cut tumors off the spinal cord. Lasers are used more often in ophthalmology than in any other field of medicine. In ophthalmology, lasers have been used for over thirty years and are used on a routine basis. In 1963, just three years after the invention of the laser, one was first used to treat a diseased eye.

Lasers are used to treat several different types of eye problems, and several different kinds of lasers are used. Argon lasers are used to treat complications of diabetes within the eye, as well as to lower the pressure inside the eye in cases of glaucoma. Krypton lasers are used to seal off dangerous new blood vessels that can grow under the retina. YAG (yttrium-aluminum-garnet) lasers are used to vaporize cloudy membranes that can form inside the eye after cataract surgery. Hundreds of thousands of patients undergo these different laser procedures every year.

THE HISTORY OF
LASER VISION CORRECTION

Laser vision correction is the intricate merging of several distinct technologies: computers, lasers, and refractive surgery techniques. Many, many people have been involved in the refinement of each of these separate aspects, and many other people have been instrumental in putting all of these pieces together.

The excimer laser, used in laser vision correction, was developed in 1976 at IBM, with the hope that it would be useful in etching computer chips. In 1982, an IBM researcher, R. Srinivasan, Ph.D., was testing the excimer laser on biological material, such as hair. Dr. Srinivasan demonstrated that smooth grooves could be reproducibly etched into a human hair without burning or otherwise damaging the surrounding portions of the hair strand.

Stephen Trokel, M.D., an ophthalmologist at Columbia University in New York City, saw a picture of the etched hair and visited Dr. Srinivasan at his IBM laboratory in 1983. There, Dr. Trokel performed laboratory studies and confirmed that a very important technological breakthrough had occurred.

From that point on, much research and development began to occur all over the world, most extensively in the United States.

The first excimer laser treatment was performed in 1985 by Dr. Theo Seiler of Germany. Dr. Seiler used the laser to make an incision in the cornea, similar to the incisons made in radial keratotomy (RK). Animal tests quickly confirmed that the excimer laser could more optimally reshape the cornea by removing a thin layer of tissue from the cornea's surface, a technique known as photorefractive keratectomy (PRK).

In 1987, Francis L'Esperance, M.D., of Columbia University became the first doctor to use the excimer laser on a human being for PRK. One of the first patients had cancer inside his eye and was going to have the eye removed. The patient agreed to allow his eye to undergo this experimental treatment before it was removed. In 1988, the first fully sighted eye underwent PRK treatment for the correction of nearsightedness. This was performed by Marguerite McDonald, M.D., at Louisiana State Univeristy.

Doctors have utilized corneal flaps in eye surgery since the 1970s. Lasik is a combination of this flap technology and the excimer laser technology, and this was first accomplished by an ophthalmologist from Crete, Ioannis Pallikaris, M.D. The first experiments combining corneal flaps and laser treatment, in 1989, were performed on blind volunteers. By 1991, Dr. Pallikaris began to perform Lasik on seeing eyes. Lasik was first performed in the United States in 1991 on an investigational basis.

The United States Food and Drug Administration (FDA) approved the laser for widespread treatment within the United States in 1995. Originally, only PRK was performed, but within two years many doctors were performing Lasik as well. At first, only nearsightedness could be treated, but the lasers were quickly adapted to treat astigmatism, and then farsightedness.

As the high degree of safety and effectiveness became apparent, doctors in many countries across Europe, Asia, and South America began performing laser vision correction.

Many important refinements in the techniques quickly occurred, resulting in improved results. Treatment zones were made larger to improve night vision. Trackers originally developed to help shoot down incoming missiles were adapted to laser eye treatment, allowing the laser beam to follow the eye as it rapidly moves. Improved diagnostic techniques enable doctors to more accurately separate those who can safely and effectively undergo the treatment and those who are not appropriate candidates. Laser manufacturers from the United States, Germany, Switzerland, and Japan have continued to introduce innovations to make the experience easier and the results even better.

In 2003, a major advance occurred with the introduction of custom wavefront treatments. Originally developed by astronomers to counteract the distortions of the atmosphere when visualizing distant stars, wave-

front techniques permit the correction of subtle irregularities in vision that are untreatable with glasses or soft
contact lenses.

Today, laser vision correction is one of the most
commonly performed medical treatments in the world.
Millions of laser vision correction treatments are performed each year, and laser vision correction is available in every advanced country in the world.

||||||||||||||||||||||||||||

WHO MONITORS
THIS TECHNIQUE?
THE ROLE OF THE FDA

The Food and Drug Administration (FDA) is the agency of the U.S. government responsible for ensuring that drugs and medical products are safe and effective. Each manufacturer's excimer laser must be approved as safe and effective by the FDA before it can be used routinely in the United States. Most countries around the world have similar agencies that investigate and monitor medical products, but none is as thorough and demanding as the FDA.

Before 1938, new drugs or medical devices could be used in the United States without any study or approval by the government. If significant complications occurred, then the federal government would investigate the product and, if necessary, remove the product from the market. The Food, Drug and Cosmetic Act of 1938 requires manufacturers to test drugs and medical products thoroughly before they sell them to the general public. Although this process significantly delays the introduction of new drugs or devices, it does prevent most dangerous products from reaching the marketplace.

How does the FDA decide whether a product is safe? First, the product is tested on animals, and if the results are favorable, carefully controlled human tests conducted in the United States will follow. Only small numbers of people are tested at first, and if the results are favorable, larger numbers of people are tested. The FDA approves a drug or product only if it is convinced that adequate numbers of people have been tested and that these tests have been carefully conducted and their results adequately studied.

In the case of vision correction lasers, each manufacturer conducts large-scale FDA studies. As advances are made in laser design, each substantially different or improved device must first be tested under the auspices of the FDA. The original small-scale FDA studies were begun in 1988 and were performed on blind or partially sighted eyes. Large-scale testing involving several thousand patients began in the United States in 1991, and the mandatory two-year follow-up period ended in 1994. Currently, many companies are involved in FDA-supervised tests of refractive eye laser technology. At least six laser companies have completed the rigorous FDA tests and achieved FDA approval.

||||||||||||||||||||||||||||

FIVE IMPORTANT
TESTS—AND WHAT
THEY MEAN

During the course of your presurgical evaluation, your doctor will perform tests on your eyes to assess your suitability for laser vision correction. These tests include corneal topography, low-light pupil size, corneal thickness, refraction, and wavefront.

MAPPING THE CORNEA:
CORNEAL TOPOGRAPHY

Corneal topography is a fascinating technique that uses a computer and a video camera to create a detailed map of the surface of the cornea. Over five thousand individual points on the cornea are measured within a fraction of a second. The computer then generates a map of the entire cornea, using different shades to represent different curvatures. Subtle variations in the curvature of the cornea can be detected. Corneal topography

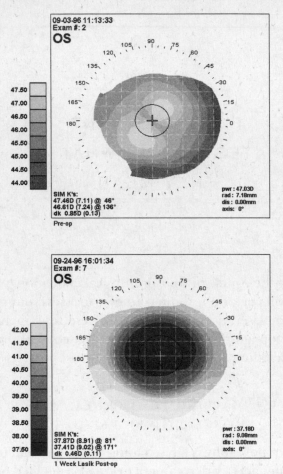

These corneal topography maps show the effects of the laser treatment. The computer map at the top was taken prior to the laser procedure and shows an eye with moderate nearsightedness and astigmatism. Each shade of gray represents a different degree of curvature. The laser treatment alters the cornea curvature, as evidenced by the map at the bottom. These curvature changes are much too small to be appreciated without these sophisticated mapping techniques.

maps help the doctor to evaluate the cornea prior to laser treatment.

For example, a map taken during the presurgical evaluation will sometimes reveal abnormal curvatures of the cornea, such as the condition of keratoconus, that make Lasik unadvisable. After the laser treatment, your doctor will often use corneal topography to follow your course of healing.

Low-Light Pupil Size

The pupil, which is the black part in the center of the eye, is the opening through which light enters the back area of the eye. When we are in bright light, the pupil becomes smaller to let in less light, and when we are in a dark area, our pupil becomes larger to let in more light.

Just as some people have larger hands or necks, some people have pupils that are larger than average, particularly in low-light conditions. This may cause problems with contact lenses and also after laser vision correction, especially if the pupil gets much larger than the portion of the cornea that is treated. In such a situation, some of the light rays passing through the pupil will have passed through untreated portions of the cornea, and these light rays will not have the proper focus. When these light rays mix with the properly focused light rays, especially in low-light conditions, the result may be nighttime glare, halos around lights, or blurriness at night.

People with extremely large pupils are at a greater risk of developing these side effects. Additional factors, such as very large corrections, also increase the likelihood of developing halos or blurriness at night. Fortunately, advances in technology have dramatically lessened the side effect of noticeable nighttime halos or glare. Mild halos during the initial weeks or months are common, but typically return to the level present prior to laser treatment, or even better, by three months.

CORNEAL THICKNESS

The cornea is composed of many layers of fibers, which combine to create the strength needed for the cornea to maintain its shape. In the Lasik procedure, a flap is made and tissue is then removed beneath the flap. It is important that enough tissue is left undisturbed to ensure the structural integrity of the cornea.

Prior to performing Lasik, your doctor will measure the thickness of your cornea and will calculate whether your cornea is thick enough to perform laser vision correction. If your cornea is not thick enough for Lasik, you can usually have PRK. PRK does not involve making a flap and can usually be performed on corneas that are too thin for Lasik.

REFRACTION

A person has nearsightedness, farsightedness, or astigmatism because the light is not being focused accurately onto the retina at the back of the eye. The careful measurement of the exact correction needed for clear focusing is known as a "refraction." The refraction is the most important measurement, because it determines exactly how much the cornea must be altered to achieve excellent vision.

A refraction is performed through a technique of trial and error by asking the patient to compare different lenses placed in front of the eye. Patients often worry that they are giving inaccurate responses, but the doctor will go over the same choices again and again to ensure consistent responses.

In this high-tech field, the trial and error method of refraction seems rather archaic. In fact, lasers can be used to perform refractions, but the laser measurements are less useful than the "which is better, one or two" method. The reason for this is quite interesting: Lasers are very accurate in measuring the eye itself, but what is more important is how you are interpreting what you are seeing. Therefore, a technique which involves the patient comparing and providing feedback is actually more useful than a purely mechanical measurement of the eyeball.

Usually, as a double check, the refraction is repeated after the eye has been dilated, during which the focusing muscles inside the eye have been temporarily inactivated. If there is any uncertainty about the accuracy, the refraction can be repeated a third or fourth time.

WAVEFRONT

In addition to the focusing errors correctable with glasses or contact lenses—nearsightedness, farsightedness, and astigmatism—the eyes have other, more subtle imperfections. These imperfections, if significant, can affect the quality of the vision, especially in lower contrast or lower light situations.

Wavefront technology enables doctors to measure and treat these subtle imperfections, which are known as higher order aberrations. Wavefront technology has significantly improved the quality of vision that is achieved with laser vision correction. Often, a patient will see better after laser vision correction, without any glasses or contacts, than they could before the treatment with glasses or contact lenses.

Wavefront measurements are obtained in just a few seconds. "There was really nothing to it," explained Marcia. "I looked into a machine, heard a few clicks, and the technician said the measurement was finished. Nothing touched my eye. It couldn't have been easier."

||||||||||||||||||||||||||||

ALTERNATIVES TO
LASER VISION CORRECTION

In addition to laser vision correction, several other techniques are currently available to treat nearsightedness, farsightedness, and astigmatism. All these treatments share the same goal as laser vision correction—to modify the focusing power of the eye in a predictable, safe, and permanent manner. Intraocular lenses—lenses placed inside the eye—are often recommended for patients who are not appropriate for laser vision correction. Conductive keratoplasty and corneal rings are currently used to correct focusing errors in selected situations. RK and ALK are now seldom used, having been replaced by more accurate techniques. Orthokeratology is a nonsurgical method to temporarily treat some focusing errors. And, of course, glasses and contact lenses are always available.

Intraocular Lenses

Intraocular lenses are tiny plastic lenses inserted inside the eye, behind the cornea. These lenses bend the incoming light rays and can correct nearsightedness, farsightedness, and astigmatism. Intraocular lenses work like contact lenses, except that they are inside the eye and are permanent.

Intraocular implants have been used successfully for many years to replace the crystalline lens of the eye when it turns cloudy—forming a cataract—and has to be removed. Cataract removal with an intraocular lens implant is a very common procedure: over one million are performed every year in the United States. More recently, people without cataracts have begun to have lens replacement treatment for their nearsightedness or farsightedness. The procedure is identical to the cataract removal procedure and is referred to as clear lens extraction or natural lens replacement.

Intraocular implants may also be placed without removing the eye's natural crystalline lens. These are known as phakic lenses or phakic implants. Some phakic lenses are placed in front of the iris (the colored part of the eye) and are known as anterior chamber implants. These are visible in front of the iris when you look carefully into the eye. Others are placed behind the iris and are referred to as posterior chamber implants.

Implant surgery is considered more invasive than laser vision correction, because the treatment involves entering the inside of the eye. Also, a foreign body is placed into the eye. Phakic lens insertion, which leaves the natural lens in the eye, is less invasive than natural lens replacement. However, with phakic lenses, the implant is near important structures in the eye and in rare cases can cause damage to the natural lens or the cornea.

Phakic implants are an option for people of any age who are too nearsighted to have laser vision correction. Natural lens replacement is a good option for people over sixty who have higher amounts of farsightedness. Natural lens replacement remains controversial for patients with large amounts of nearsightedness due to an increased risk of retinal detachment complications.

CONDUCTIVE KERATOPLASTY (CK)

Conductive keratoplasty, also known as CK, uses radio frequency energy to alter the shape of the cornea. CK can be used to decrease farsightedness or to create monovision, in which one eye is adjusted for near to lessen the need for up-close reading glasses.

The CK procedure is quick and almost pain-free. A series of eight focal treatments are placed in the periphery of the cornea. This causes the central cornea to steepen. CK has not gained the same level of popularity as laser vision correction. It is only appropriate for a small number of patients. The vision after CK takes longer to stabilize than after Lasik. If the initial result is not as precise as intended, a touch-up CK can usually be performed, but rarely the touch-up must be performed with laser vision correction.

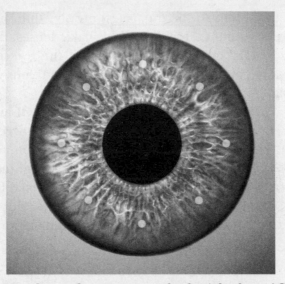

Conductive keratoplasty treatment for farsightedness (CK). A series of focal treatments in the peripheral cornea causes the central cornea to steepen.

CORNEAL RINGS (INTACS)

Corneal rings (also known as Intacs) are small pieces of plastic that are embedded in the edge of the cornea. The arc-shaped rings make the central portion of the cornea flatter, decreasing the amount of nearsightedness. Corneal rings are available to treat only low amounts of nearsightedness and cannot be used for farsightedness, astigmatism, or larger amounts of nearsightedness.

By using rings of varying thicknesses, different amounts of nearsightedness can be corrected. However, corneal rings are made in only a limited number of

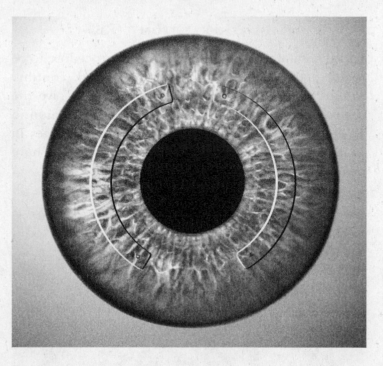

The corneal ring technique places two thin pieces of plastic in the edge of the cornea, which causes the central cornea to change shape.

thicknesses, so they can only be used for very specific corrections. If the visual result is not ideal, or if the eye changes in the future, the corneal rings can be removed, but there might not be another ring that is appropriate to correct your vision. In contrast, laser vision correction is available for a wide range of focusing errors and is easily adjustable with re-treatments.

Radial Keratotomy (RK)

Radial keratotomy was the first surgical procedure to be widely used to correct nearsightedness and, contrary to most people's understanding, does not involve the use of a laser. RK was invented in the Soviet Union in 1973 and was first performed in the United States in 1978. Over one million people around the world have been treated with RK.

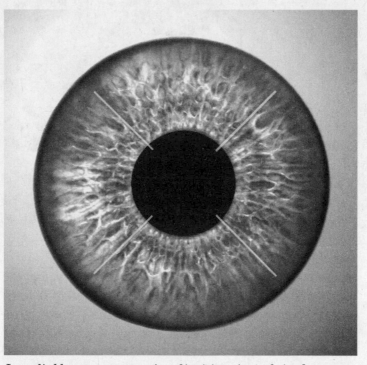

In radial keratotomy, a series of incisions is made in the cornea, causing the central cornea to flatten.

In RK, the doctor makes a series of incisions in the periphery of the cornea. This increases the corneal curvature slightly where the incisions are made and decreases the curvature in the central portion of the cornea. The incisions are made in a radiating pattern, like the spokes on a bicycle wheel. By varying the number, length, depth, and location of these incisions, different amounts of nearsightedness can be corrected.

Although patient satisfaction with RK was high, RK has been largely replaced by laser vision correction and is seldom used today.

Automated Lamellar Keratoplasty (ALK)

Performed from the 1970s until the mid-1990s, ALK was the forerunner to Lasik. In ALK, the front layers of the cornea were separated and folded away, creating a flap, similar to the Lasik procedure today. In ALK, the flap-making device was then used a second time to remove a small disc of cornea from under the flap, causing the central cornea to flatten and lessening nearsightedness. In Lasik, the tissue under the flap is instead reshaped using a laser, which is much more precise.

ALK has been completely replaced by Lasik and is not performed anymore. In fact, ALK was never very popular because the second part of the procedure, removing the disc of tissue, was not adequately precise. However, without ALK we would probably not have Lasik today. Lasik is a combination of the flap technique of ALK with the precision of the excimer laser—a truly remarkable combination.

Because ALK has been performed since the 1970s, we have a long track record showing the safety of making corneal flaps. This is very important: Because of ALK, we know that there are no long-term safety problems from making corneal flaps!

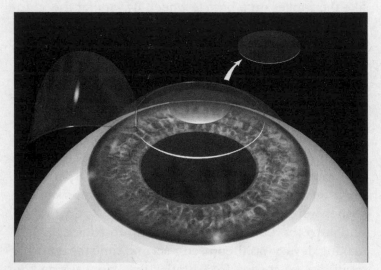

In automated lamellar keratoplasty for nearsightedness, the outer cornea is folded back and a small piece of tissue is removed.

ORTHOKERATOLOGY

Orthokeratology is not a surgical correction. Rather, it involves the use, over a course of months, of progressively flatter contact lenses to reduce the curvature of the cornea. After completing the course of treatment, the patient can see clearly for many hours without con-

tact lenses or glasses. The patient continues to wear retainer contact lenses from two to seven times a week,
usually while sleeping. Thus, successful orthokeratology
results in the patient not needing contact lenses while
awake, but wearing retainer contact lenses while asleep.
If the patient stops wearing the retainer contact lens, his
or her eye reverts to its original nearsightedness within
one week.

Orthokeratology can temporarily correct mild nearsightedness, up to about 3 diopters, and works best for
people needing 2 diopters or less of correction. It is not
successful in all patients, because some patients develop
a distortion of the cornea and have to discontinue treatment.

Orthokeratology is an option for patients with
mild or very mild nearsightedness who may be able
to tolerate contact lenses well but prefer not to wear
them in public and do not want to have laser vision
correction treatment. People in certain occupations,
such as policemen, firemen, or flight attendants, may
use orthokeratology to pass their vision test require-
ments.

GLASSES AND CONTACT LENSES

Of course, most people have their nearsightedness, farsightedness, and astigmatism corrected with glasses or
contact lenses. Although it may be inconvenient to wear
glasses or contact lenses, they do provide excellent vision in most cases. If you are satisfied using glasses or
contact lenses, then there is no need for other forms of

treatment. You should consider other treatments only if your glasses or contact lenses are uncomfortable or inconvenient or if you want good vision without glasses and contact lenses for personal or occupational reasons.

NO MORE READING GLASSES?

The most common focusing problem in the world is not nearsightedness, farsightedness, or astigmatism. Presbyopia (which means "old vision") is by far the most common focusing problem, because it affects every person beginning around age forty to fifty. Objects that are close to us require more focusing strength than objects that are far away. In young people, the crystalline lens changes shape (and thereby its focusing strength), depending on whether you are focusing on something in the distance or up close. This ability to change the focus from distance to near is known as accommodation. As we approach the age of forty to fifty, the crystalline lens gets stiffer and we begin to lose our accommodation. The age-related loss of accommodation, which occurs in every person, is known as presbyopia.

Unfortunately, none of the techniques used to treat nearsightedness, farsightedness, or astigmatism also solves the problem of presbyopia.

People deal with presbyopia in several ways. The most common way of dealing with presbyopia is to use reading glasses, bifocals, or trifocals. Some people with presbyopia choose to have monovision, in which one eye is adjusted for distance and the other is adjusted for near. Monovision can be created with glasses, contact lenses, laser vision correction, or any of the other surgical treatments discussed earlier. Some people over forty-five years old with mild nearsightedness, whose eyes are thereby naturally adjusted for near vision, simply remove their distance glasses to see clearly up close. However, these nearsighted people who also have presbyopia are unable to see clearly up close when their distance glasses or contact lenses are on.

Several techniques are now being tested that may provide relief for presbyopia.

Natural lens replacement with bifocal implants is one treatment for presbyopia that is already being used, although only in special circumstances. In this technique, which is similar to a cataract surgery, the crystalline lens inside the eye is removed and replaced with a plastic lens that has bifocal focusing abilities. The treatment is quick—requiring about fifteen minutes. Natural lens replacement is more invasive than laser vision correction, because it involves entering the inside of the eye, and is subject to more and greater risks. Also, some people are not satisfied with the quality of the distance or near vision obtained with the current versions of implants.

Corneal inlays are very thin pieces of plastic that are placed in the center of the cornea. In one design, a reading prescription is incorporated into a very small inlay placed in the center of the line of vision. In another design, a thin inlay with a 1.6 millimeter central hole is inserted. This increases the depth of field, enabling a person with presbyopia to regain their near vision without the need for reading glasses.

Scleral expansion bands (SEBs) are four small pieces of plastic that are inserted into the white portion of the eye (the sclera). SEBs appear to improve the ability of people with presbyopia to read clearly up close, eliminating the need for reading glasses, without affecting the distance vision. SEBs are currently being tested for safety and effectiveness by the FDA.

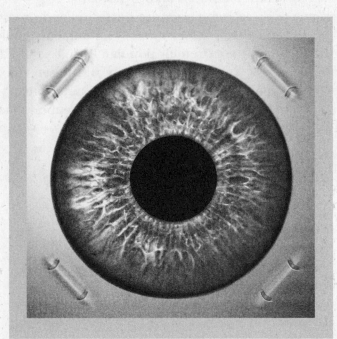

Four scleral expansion bands are placed in the white part of the eye, eliminating the need for reading glasses.

Another technique, known as anterior ciliary sclerostomy, is also being examined as a means of correcting presbyopia. Anterior ciliary sclerostomy involves making radiating incisions in the sclera. These incisions are similar to the incisions used in radial keratotomy (RK), except in RK the incisions are placed in the cornea. Some companies are testing making the incisions with a laser, as well as placing small pieces of plastic into the incisions to magnify the results.

Bifocal laser vision correction is also being tested. Thus far, it has met with only limited success, but much research on this method is taking place.

If any of these techniques are perfected and proven to be safe and effective over time, the treatments would most likely become extremely popular. People would be able to correct their distance acuity with laser vision correction and then correct their age-limited near vision as well. Until then, we will have to rely upon reading glasses and monovision.

||||||||||||||||||||||||||

AFTERWORD

|||||||||||||||||||||||||||||||

MY OWN EXPERIENCE
AS A PATIENT

began wearing glasses when I was twelve years old. Although I could see very well with them, I never liked the way I looked in glasses. Growing up in Florida, I loved to swim, but I couldn't see very well when I took my glasses off. Playing sports with glasses was often a problem, because my glasses would become foggy, sweaty, or would get knocked around.

I started wearing contact lenses during high school. These were much better than glasses for me. They didn't fog or get wet in the rain, and I had much better peripheral vision. Also, the contacts didn't cause the distortions that I always had with my glasses. My early contacts were hard lenses, and it did take a few miserable weeks to adjust to them. Occasionally a piece of dust would get under the lens and it felt like my eye was on fire.

During medical school at the age of twenty-two, I started to wear soft lenses, and these were better still.

The soft lenses were comfortable from the first day, and I could wear them almost all day long. However, after a long day of working in the hospital, my eyes would usually be very sore, and I would need to take the contacts out. Hopefully I had my glasses nearby. Some days my eyes would be so sore that I couldn't wear the contacts at all.

Wouldn't it be great, I often thought, if I didn't need these glasses or contacts? Growing up, I viewed my nearsightedness and astigmatism as my biggest handicap, so it wasn't surprising that after completing medical school, I specialized in ophthalmology and concentrated my practice on correcting vision focusing problems.

Day after day, year after year, my patients would tell me that correcting their nearsightedness and astigmatism was one of the best things that had ever happened to them. I treated my own brother and many of my closest friends, in each case with fantastic results. However, because of my relatively high amount of nearsightedness, I was never an excellent candidate for radial keratotomy, the only technique then available, which was incredibly frustrating. I was, however, a good candidate for laser vision correction, so when the procedure became available in the United States, I decided to have it myself.

I chose to have the Lasik technique because of the faster visual recovery.

I knew that there was no guarantee that I would obtain a perfect correction, but I also knew that there was a high probability that I would see well enough to do away with my glasses and contacts for most activities. Because I was over forty years old, I had been noticing some difficulty with near vision, though I hadn't yet started to use reading glasses or bifocals. I knew that laser treatment would not solve this problem and that in the next several years I would begin to need reading glasses.

During the preoperative examination, my eyes were examined and my nearsightedness and astigmatism were measured. Corneal topography was performed. I was asked to read and sign a long document, which explained the technique, including what it could do and what could go wrong. The doctor also discussed the more common complications with me. Although I had gone over this with my own patients thousands of times, I still listened very carefully.

In 1996, when my Lasik procedure was performed, it was standard practice to treat one eye on one day and the other eye the next day. This is how I was treated. Today, almost all people have both eyes treated on the same day, which is considerably more convenient. The procedure itself was very easy. First, my eye was washed out and numbing drops were put in. After lying down on the table, a speculum was placed in my eyelids to keep them open. All I could really see were several very bright lights. The doctor then created the thin flap, which didn't hurt and took only a few seconds. I was then asked to look at a blinking light, and I heard the clicking noise of the laser. Again, there was no pain. During the course of the treatment, the blinking light became blurry and changed shape, but I was still able to look at it. The doctor then rinsed the eye and folded the flap back into place. The whole treatment had taken less than five minutes.

A few minutes later, a stinging feeling began in the eye. I didn't take any pain medicine, because the stinging wasn't very bad, but someone else might have wanted to take a mild pain pill. I took a nap, and after three or four hours, the stinging feeling went away. I put in the first of the eyedrops, which I was told to continue using for a week.

The morning after my Lasik, I was stunned by how good my vision was. It wasn't perfect, but it was very, very good. It had improved so much in such a short time! I was able to drive myself the day after the procedure. Reading was a little strained during the first several weeks, and my vision would fluctuate somewhat during the day. During the first several weeks, I also experienced glare and halos around lights, but this gradually receded.

I returned to work three days after my procedure. After two weeks I felt very comfortable with my vision and resumed performing surgery.

During the next few months, my vision gradually became sharper. There was still some fluctuation; there were some times when the vision seemed sharper, and other times when it was less precise. During the first several months, my vision was poor in dim light, and I experienced mild double vision with the left eye. These problems resolved after three to four months.

I am now able to work, drive, play sports, and go to movies without needing any glasses or contacts for my distance vision. My eyes are a lot less irritated now that I don't wear contacts; they are whiter and less sensitive to the sun. I can see well when I wake up in the morning, and swimming and other sports have become a lot more fun. I don't have to bother with all those contact lens solutions and I don't have to worry about having an extra pair of glasses available. My clear vision is now part of me, instead of something I would put on and take off.

When I had my Lasik treatment, my children, Bryce and Jocelyn, were young, and they were actually very disappointed. They loved to give me a big kiss each morning, then pull off my glasses and throw them around. But suddenly there weren't any glasses to play around with anymore!

My Lasik procedure was more than a decade ago and I have enjoyed great distance vision all these years. The hassles of glasses and contact lenses are really just an old memory. Since I am now over 50, I have started using reading glasses, and as I get older I have noticed that I do need them more and more. But I know that I would have needed the reading glasses anyway, only I would have needed glasses or contacts for distance vision as well. Now I wake up in the morning, walk around, drive, and play sports without any glasses or contact lenses at all, and I could not be any happier with my vision.

APPENDIXES

OTHER SOURCES
OF INFORMATION

American Academy of Ophthalmology
P.O. Box 7424
655 Beach Street
San Francisco, CA 94109
www.aao.org

American Optometric Association
243 N. Lindbergh Boulevard
St. Louis, MO 63141
www.aoa.org

American Society of Cataract and Refractive Surgery
4000 Legato Road, Suite 850
Fairfax, VA 22033
www.ascrs.org

Council for Refractive Surgery Quality Assurance
8543 Everglade Drive
Sacramento, CA 95826-3616
www.usaeyes.org

Food and Drug Administration (FDA)
5600 Fishers Lane (HFE-99)
Rockville, MD 20852
www.fda.gov/cdrh/LASIK

GLOSSARY

It is hard to understand a technical subject such as laser vision correction without using specialized words.

Here are definitions of some of the terms used in refractive surgery and in this book.

aberration: an imperfection in the vision, usually divided into lower order and higher order aberrations.

ablation: removal of tissue, for example, from the front surface of the cornea.

accommodation: the ability of the eye to change focus from distance to midrange to near; the loss of accommodation is known as presbyopia.

AK: (see astigmatic keratotomy).

ALK: (see automated lamellar keratoplasty).

amblyopia (lazy eye): a condition in which the eye structure is normal but the processing of visual information limits the visual acuity.

ametropia: a condition of imprecise focus, such as near-sightedness or farsightedness.

anterior ciliary sclerostomy: an experimental technique to treat presbyopia.

argon laser: a type of laser commonly used to treat glaucoma, retinal, and diabetic eye diseases.

astigmatic keratotomy (AK): a variation of radial keratotomy, in which incisions are made into the surface of the cornea to correct astigmatism.

astigmatism: asymmetrical focus of the light rays.

automated lamellar keratoplasty (ALK): a procedure for correcting nearsightedness or farsightedness in which a layer of cornea is cut, and sometimes an additional layer is removed.

axis: the direction of the astigmatism.

bilateral: pertaining to two sides; pertaining to both eyes.

Bowman's layer: the layer of the cornea lying directly beneath the epithelium.

cataracts: a clouding of the crystalline lens of the eye; if severe, surgical removal of the crystalline lens is needed.

central islands: a complication of excimer laser treatment in which the central corneal surface becomes raised.

CK: (see conductive keratoplasty).

clear lens extraction; clear lens replacement: the removal and replacement of the crystalline lens of the eye to treat nearsightedness or farsightedness; the same as natural lens replacement.

coma: an imperfection in vision in which there is asymmetrical focusing of light.

conductive keratoplasty: a technique to correct farsightedness that uses radio frequency energy; same as radio frequency keratoplasty.

contrast sensitivity: a measure of visual ability, specifically the ability to distinguish details under varying degrees of contrast.

cornea: the transparent tissue at the front of the eye.

corneal ring: a small plastic device placed in the cornea to correct nearsightedness; also known as the ICR, intrastomal corneal ring, or Intacs.

corneal topography: a computer-assisted technique for measuring the surface contours of the cornea.

crystalline lens: the hard tissue located just behind the iris, which focuses light rays.

decentration: a complication during excimer laser surgery in which the tissue is removed off center.

diopter: the measurement of a lens's ability to focus light rays. One diopter of focusing ability will focus parallel rays of light at one meter.

ectasia: (see keratectasia).

emmetropia: the normal condition of the eye in which the light rays focus on the retina.

endothelium: the innermost layer of cells in the cornea. The endothelium is responsible for pumping fluid out of the cornea, which is necessary to maintain corneal clarity.

epikeratophakia: a discontinued procedure for the correction of nearsightedness in which a lens is sewn onto the surface of the cornea.

Epi-Lasik: a version of PRK in which the epithelium is removed with a dull keratome.

epithelium: the thin, jellylike layer of cells on the surface of the cornea. In PRK, this tissue is removed and grows back in about three days.

excimer laser: an argon-fluorine gas laser that produces an ultraviolet beam used to remove corneal tissue accurately.

farsightedness (hyperopia): a focusing error in which the light rays are focused behind the retina. This results when the cornea and the crystalline lens together have too little focusing power for the length of the eye.

FDA (Food and Drug Administration): an agency of the federal government that monitors new medical devices and drugs.

flap and zap: the nickname for laser in-situ keratomileusis (LASIK), a procedure in which a flap is made in the cornea and excimer laser energy is then applied to tissue inside the cornea.

glaucoma: a disease characterized by abnormally high pressure within the eye.

haze: a complication of PRK treatment in which the cornea develops cloudiness.

hexagonal keratotomy: a discontinued procedure for the correction of farsightedness, involving making cuts into the cornea in the shape of a hexagon.

higher order aberrations: imperfections in vision that cannot be corrected with glasses. The most common higher order aberrations are coma and spherical aberration.

HOA: (see higher order aberrations).

holmium laser: a laser previously used to correct farsightedness. This technique is no longer performed.

hyperopia (farsightedness): a focusing error in which the light rays are focused behind the retina. This results when the cornea and the crystalline lens together have too little focusing power for the length of the eye.

ICR (intrastromal corneal ring): a small plastic device placed in the cornea to correct nearsightedness; also known as corneal ring or Intacs.

informed consent: the legal process whereby a patient receives and acknowledges the risks, benefits, and alternatives to a medical procedure.

Intacs: the ICR (intrastromal corneal ring) manufactured by Addition Technology.

IntraLase: the first company to manufacture a laser keratome.

intraocular implants: plastic lenses placed in front of or behind the iris to correct nearsightedness, farsightedness, or astigmatism.

intraocular lenses: (see intraocular implants).

intrastromal: within the cornea, as opposed to on the surface of the cornea.

intrastromal corneal ring (ICR): a small plastic ring used to correct nearsightedness. The ring is placed inside the edge of the cornea.

intrastromal lens: a clear lens placed within the cornea for correction of focusing abnormalities.

iris: the visible colored tissue inside the eye.

irregular astigmatism: irregular curvature of the cornea.

keratectasia: a bulging of the cornea after laser vision correction, similar to keratoconus.

kerato-: of, or pertaining to, the cornea. From the Greek word for "cornea."

keratoconus: a disease of the cornea in which the central cornea becomes thinner and irregularly shaped.

keratome: an instrument used in creating the flap in the Lasik technique.

keratomileusis: an abandoned surgical procedure to correct nearsightedness in which a piece of the cornea is removed, reshaped, and reattached.

keratoplasty: surgical alteration of the cornea.

krypton laser: a type of laser used to treat retinal eye disease.

lamellar keratoplasty: a procedure for correcting nearsightedness or farsightedness in which a layer of cornea is cut, and sometimes an additional layer is cut and removed.

Lasek (laser assisted epithelial keratomileusis): a version of PRK in which the epithelium is replaced after laser treatment is complete.

laser: a device that creates a beam of light that is perfectly synchronized and of the same wavelength.

laser in-situ keratomileusis (Lasik): a procedure in which a flap is made in the cornea and excimer laser energy is then applied to tissue inside the cornea; also known as "flap and zap."

laser thermal keratoplasty (LTK): an abandoned procedure that uses a laser to heat portions of the cornea, resulting in the correction of farsightedness.

Lasik: (see laser in-situ keratomileusis).

lazy eye: (see amblyopia).

lens: a device that focuses light rays.

LOA: (see lower order aberrations).

lower order aberrations: imperfections in the vision cor-

rectable with glasses—nearsightedness, farsightedness, and astigmatism.

LTK: (see laser thermal keratoplasty).

micron: one millionth of a meter, or a thousandth of a
millimeter; equivalent to about 39 millionths of an
inch (also known as "micrometer").

microkeratome: (see keratome).

monovision: adjusting the vision in one eye for distance
and in the other eye for near vision. This is an alternative to reading glasses and can be accomplished
with contact lenses or with refractive surgery.

myopia (nearsightedness): a focusing error in which the
light rays are focused in front of the retina. This results when the cornea and the crystalline lens together have too much focusing power for the
length of the eye.

nearsightedness: (see myopia).

natural lens replacement: the removal and replacement
of the crystalline lens of the eye to treat nearsightedness or farsightedness; the same as clear lens replacement.

off-label: the use of an FDA-approved drug or medical
device in a way that has not been explicitly approved by the FDA.

optic nerve: the nerve behind the eye that transmits
visual information from the eye to the brain.

optical zone: in radial keratotomy, the area of the central cornea in which incisions are not placed.

orthokeratology: a technique for temporarily decreasing the curvature of the cornea using contact
lenses.

overcorrection: a complication of laser vision correction in which the eye reacts more than anticipated.

pachymeter: a device that measures the thickness of the cornea, usually by ultrasound.

PERK (prospective evaluation of radial keratotomy) study: a study funded by the National Institutes of Health that studied 435 patients who had radial keratotomy surgery beginning in 1982.

phakic: referring to the natural crystalline lens of the eye.

phakic intraocular implants: lenses placed into the eye in addition to the natural crystalline lens.

photorefractive keratectomy (PRK): an excimer laser procedure to correct nearsightedness, farsightedness, or astigmatism in which tissue is removed from the surface of the cornea.

phototherapeutic keratectomy (PTK): an excimer laser surgical procedure in which tissue is removed from the surface of the cornea to remove scars and other irregularities.

presbyopia: the gradual loss of the ability to adjust the eye's focus that is a normal part of the aging process. This results in a loss of the ability to adjust focus from distant to nearby objects.

PRK: (see photorefractive keratectomy).

progressive hyperopia: a complication of radial keratotomy in which a progressive flattening of the cornea occurs months or years after the procedure.

PTK: (see phototherapeutic keratectomy).

pupil: the black opening in the iris that gets larger or smaller depending on the amount of light entering the eye.

radial keratotomy (RK): a surgical procedure for correcting nearsightedness, in which small incisions are made in the surface of the cornea.

radio frequency keratoplasty: a technique to correct farsightedness that uses radio frequency energy; same as conductive keratoplasty.

refraction: in ophthalmology, measuring the focus of the eye, usually by placing multiple test lenses in front of the eye.

refractive error: an inaccuracy in the focusing ability of the eye; includes nearsightedness, farsightedness, and astigmatism.

refractive surgery: the surgical correction of refractive errors.

regression: a complication of excimer laser surgery in which an initially favorable result changes in the direction of the original condition.

regular astigmatism: astigmatism that is symmetrical and can be corrected with glasses.

retina: the tissue in the back of the eye that receives the light rays.

RFK: (see radio frequency keratoplasty).

RK: (see radial keratotomy).

SBK: (see sub-Bowman's keratomileusis).

sclera: the white tissue that surrounds the eyeball.

scleral expansion band: a device, implanted into the white portion of the eye, that is being tested to correct presbyopia.

sclerostomy: (see anterior ciliary sclerostomy).

SEB: (see scleral expansion band).

sphere: when referring to glasses, the aspect of the lens focusing for nearsightedness or farsightedness.

spherical aberration: an irregularity in vision in which the light passing through the edges of the visual system is focused differently than the light passing through the center.

sub-Bowman's keratomileusis: Lasik treatment with a very thin flap.

thermal keratoplasty: a procedure to correct farsightedness and astigmatism in which heat is applied into the cornea; lasers are now being tested for this procedure, which is known as laser thermal keratoplasty.

topography: a computer-assisted technique for measuring the surface contours of the cornea.

transepithelial: a variation of photorefractive keratectomy in which the laser is used to remove the epithelium, the thin layer of cells on the surface of the cornea.

undercorrection: a complication of laser vision correction in which the eye responds less than anticipated.

visual acuity: the ability of the eye to resolve visual detail.

visual cortex: the area of the brain that processes the visual information from the eye.

vitreous humor: the gel-like substance that fills the space between the crystalline lens and the retina.

wavefront analysis: a technique for measuring complex imperfections in vision by using light bounced off the back of the eye.

wavelength: the distance between two identical, successive parts of a wave of light; responsible for the "color" of the light.

YAG (yttrium-aluminum-garnet) laser: a laser used in ophthalmology to cut transparent membranes.

ACKNOWLEDGMENTS

A tremendous amount of work has gone into producing this book, and it would not have been possible without help from many people. First and foremost, I would like to thank my wife, Jacqueline, who has lovingly understood the countless hours that I have worked on this book before and after my normal occupation of taking care of patients. I would like to thank my office staff—most of whom have trusted me to correct their own or their spouse's vision—for bringing zest and professionalism to everything they do. Diane Shader Smith and Mark Smith provided invaluable guidance during the early phases of the book, and Alison Schneider helped add depth and warmth to the manuscript. My publisher, Claire Ferraro, and editor, Cathy Repetti, had the vision to make this project possible. My editor for the most recently revised edition, Porscha Burke, has been extremely helpful and wonderful to work with. Most of all, I would like to thank my many patients who read the manuscript; your comments helped bring clarity and completeness to this book.

INDEX

ABOUT THE AUTHOR

ANDREW I. CASTER, M.D., F.A.C.S., has performed almost thirty thousand vision correction procedures. Dr.
Caster is a graduate of Harvard College, Harvard Medical School, and the UCLA Jules Stein Eye Institute. For
more than twelve years, Dr. Caster has dedicated his
practice exclusively to laser vision correction, and he is
one of the most respected Lasik doctors in the United
States. Dr. Caster has participated in extensive clinical
research to further the advancement of Lasik treatment. Patients travel to Dr. Caster for laser vision correction from across the United States as well as from
Europe, Asia, and South America. Dr. Caster practices
in the Los Angeles, California, area with offices in Bev-
erly Hills. You can visit with Dr. Caster and the Caster
Eye Center at www.castervision.com.